MAKE IT
STOP

An insider's guide to
recovery

By David Horry

Make it Stop: An Insider's Guide to Recovery

Contents

You don't drown by falling in the water. You drown by staying there.

Edwin Louis Cole

Hope

Alcohol isn't magical. If you put a sealed, chilled, bottle of white wine in front of me then I will feel the urge to reach out and take and drink it. This urge is not imaginary; it is very real and compelling. But alcohol has no special physical, chemical or other property that can make this happen. Alcohol, sealed in a bottle, cannot direct my thoughts or desires because there is no mechanism by which this can occur, yet the urge to take it exists and it is completely real. This phenomenon goes further. If that same sealed, chilled bottle contained a liquid that *looked* like wine but was non-alcoholic then my reaction would be precisely the same. I would feel the urge to take, open and drink it even though there was no alcohol present! It isn't alcohol that controls my thoughts and actions, because I react in precisely the same way when alcohol isn't even present. It is not alcohol that makes me want to drink it; there is no mechanism by which this can happen. I manufacture the urge to drink it entirely within my own head.

My fight is not with the bottle it is with my own mind.

Popular opinion has it that alcoholics are bad people, that we are weak and make poor choices, and that our addiction is a consequence of that. But every word of that statement is incorrect. I am not broken, or a bad person, I am misled; misled by my own mind. I am not "faulty" but I *am* different. My mind does not respond to alcohol the same way as that of a normal drinker and this is why they can't understand me. Their mind recognises that it is *not* always a good or appropriate time to drink and sometimes they will be steered away from alcohol. But my mind does not work like this. My mind automatically decides that I *should* drink even when others would think it unwise to do so. I do not make bad choices, my mind never offers me a choice to make, and this difference makes me susceptible to addiction. I am not a bad or weak person but my mind responds differently to alcohol, it urges me to drink and I have no immediate or direct control over this response. Normal drinkers can choose whether or not they drink whereas in me that decision to drink has already been made, and if I am to avoid drinking then I have to actively step in and contradict it by force of will. What is different in me is that I have a susceptibility to addiction and I have activated that vulnerability, and once that susceptibility has been engaged then it accelerates under its own impetus. It is like a boulder pushed into motion down a hill. Once the boulder is moving then it gathers speed under its own momentum and the original push is no longer needed. So it is with addiction. Whether I first drank for relief from some distress or hardship, or to smother some trauma in my past, or simply because that's what everyone around me was doing, it makes no difference. I am among that part of the population that is susceptible to addiction and once I started to drink frequently then this set in place an inevitable chain of events that made the condition become progressively worse. Once it was activated then my addiction became self-fuelling and the original reason I drank became inconsequential.

I had no way of knowing that my mind was behaving differently to that of most of the population. I just carried on thinking that my drinking was a normal response to what was happening around me, but it kept getting worse. I finally reached the point where I could no longer believe the voice in my head saying that my drinking was normal, or even helpful. The accumulating evidence was that my drinking was destructive and eventually this became undeniable even to me. I had tried everything I could think of to bring my drinking under control but it could not be done. Eventually I reached the point where my drinking had become *so* damaging that it simply *had* to change and I considered the terrifying prospect that, since I couldn't control how much I drank, then I might have to stop drinking altogether.

Alcoholism isn't a simple problem, it is multi-facetted and it compounds. One problem creates another and the steadily increasing compulsion to drink is only the first of these. The consequences of sustained drinking over an extended period include a serious decline in mental well-being. Anxiety, fear, frustration, depression and hopelessness were all direct and inevitable consequences of my drinking because poor mental health and alcoholism are inseparably bound. In the same way that drinking lowered my mood, so too did the consequences of that drinking. My actions had consequences and over the years I accumulated a huge and enduring burden of guilt, shame, regret and remorse.

There is no one remedy that fixed all of my issues and I needed to attend to all aspects of the condition one by one in order to recover. This took time and it took persistence. I did not recover from addiction in hours or days; that is not how it happens. It took many months and progress was incremental rather than sudden. So if you are just starting out then prepare yourself for this; the challenge is stern, the benefits seem to come slowly, and the timescale is long. But when they came the benefits far exceeded my expectations.

Every day I continued to drink my addiction became more entrenched and harder to overcome. And while I drank then the chaos and wreckage continued and the burden of guilt, shame, regret and remorse accumulated. Every facet of my existence was falling apart. The wreckage in and around my life was growing and the burden of shame and guilt was crushing me, but I couldn't stop it. No matter what I did to control my drinking it always failed and I had tried everything I could think of. I thought about alcohol from my waking moment to the last of my consciousness... when would I get a drink, where, and how? What would it be and with whom? I was taut as a bowstring the whole time and constantly anxious, fearful, and frustrated. But there were also dark thoughts circling; I could see where this path was taking me. At some point in the future it left me in the dark, alone, with nothing, and that path was unsurvivable. The penalty for delay was that everything kept getting worse and eventually the balanced finally tipped. I finally knew that the pain of continuing exceeded the pain of stopping, and as much as it scared me I realised that "now" was the time to stop, because if I didn't then tomorrow it would be even worse. It *had* to stop. It *had* to change. But I didn't have a clue how to do it.

I had a vitally important goal, but no idea of how to achieve it. I had tried a huge number of things that didn't work, but had not found even one that kept me off the drink for more than a few days. I needed new ideas if I was to break out of this trap and in desperation I set out to find them. Other people had done this before me, so I started there; I walked into a recovery meeting.

Once I fully accepted that I had a problem and that I didn't know how to fix it myself then things changed dramatically. I had been terrified of going into a recovery meeting because of the judgement and shame I expected to come from it, but there was none of that. Instead I found compassion and understanding and I started to learn about alcoholism. I was surprised to discover that this problem isn't at all uncommon. Many people had precisely the same issues but a lot of them had managed to stop drinking and this was a revelation. I had thought that it was impossible to stop drinking, but it wasn't. There was no shortage of proof that it was possible and there was no shortage of advice on how to set about it, but what I found severely lacking was any explanation of "why". People could tell me what to do but they could not tell me why it would be effective, and that works very poorly for me. I can get keen and enthusiastic about doing something if I understand the problem and if I see how a certain action will improve it, but I am instinctively dismissive of that advice if it can't be backed up with clear evidence. When I know that an action will be effective then I will work harder at it and this was the great component I found missing in the recovery community I joined. There was plenty of advice telling me what to do, and that advice was earnestly given and probably had merit, but what was missing was any explanation of why or how it might work. "Because I say so" didn't work for me as a child and the passage of years has not improved this. If you want me to do something that I'm disinclined to then you need to explain to me *why* it is a better way, and *then* I will step into it with vigour. People were giving me advice, and those people had stopped drinking, so there was obviously something beneficial coming from the actions they suggested. But I was being invited to take that advice on faith and that isn't enough for me; I need to understand why.

I heard alcoholism often referred to as a disease and this sort of helped me but equally it sort of did not. It helped to think that this problem wasn't to do with poor choices: "it's an illness, not a weakness" they said.

But I also found "disease" to be an unsatisfactory word to describe whatever it was I had. To me diseases are something you catch, like leprosy, cholera, or yellow fever but you don't "catch" alcoholism from someone else, so I didn't like the word but it set me looking. If alcoholism was a disease then it would be known about because there were people that specialised in diseases, we call them doctors, and they're a pretty 'onto it' group of people. If alcoholism was a disease then they'd have it catalogued somehow with symptoms and treatment etc. So I looked it up, and alcoholism was indeed an illness that was well recognised by the medical establishment. It was identified, described, and studied in depth. There weren't just a few research papers on it, there were thousands, and I started to read. The more I studied then the more I understood about the causes of the condition, how it increases in complexity, and how it manifests itself. I started to understand my condition and how I had become trapped by the workings of my own brain, and when I understood those mechanisms then I could filter the advice I was being given through that knowledge. This was enormously empowering because when I understood how something would help me then my willingness to do it changed completely, and that is the purpose of this book. It identifies the things we can do to escape alcoholism and it explains why those things are effective: it changes willingness.

As I progressed through recovery I steadily learned what things helped and I tried to master those, but I didn't always succeed, and I certainly didn't succeed at my first attempt. Recovering from alcoholism is not like a test that we either pass or fail it is more like a skill we acquire, and gaining any new skill takes practise and persistence. But that experience took time to acquire and it would have helped me a lot if I'd discovered some of the things that would help me earlier. So here are sixteen things that are helpful straight away for those that are starting out now or are starting anew. These things aren't what I did when I first set out to stop drinking; they are what I did when I succeeded. Each serves a very specific purpose and the more that can be done then the easier the path becomes.

- **Don't pick up the first drink.** Do anything at all to stop you from picking up that first drink because the first drink dissolves all objections to having another. One is too many, ten is not enough.
- **Don't have alcohol in the house.** The closer you are to alcohol then the stronger is the call to drink.
- **Don't buy alcohol.** If you buy alcohol then you will drink it, all that is undecided is when. Don't buy it, and don't go into places that sell it.

- **Delay, distract, deny.** Delay having that drink until later. Do something to distract yourself until the craving passes, and deny yourself the possibility of drinking even if your resolve has collapsed.
- **Engage help.** Your doctor will be able to advise on medication for cravings and withdrawal as well as what other help is available locally.
- **Have things prepared that will occupy your mind and hands** and use them when the urge to drink is severe. Physically active things that require hand-eye coordination work well; tidy something, pack/unpack something, move stuff, weed the garden, make something, clean the inside of the car. It doesn't matter what it is but do something to fully occupy your mind and hands.
- **Radically change your daily routine** to occupy the times when you used to drink. Plan to be doing something else and somewhere else at these times.
- **If you are somewhere and you can see** drinking and feel it pulling then move away from it. Be accompanied to social events by someone who knows you're not drinking and make sure you have a way to leave if you need to.
- **Have sweet things and snacks** handy and have plenty of alcohol-free drinks ready to have a filled glass in your hand if you need it.

- **Be kind to yourself.** Give yourself "treats". Treats are rewards that your brain recognises and they will make you feel better. Alcohol is not a treat. It is not a reward it is a punishment.
- **Make deliberate time to exercise every day.** Do some things that get your heartbeat up for 15 mins or more. It makes no difference what the exercise is so walk uphill, jog, use an exercise machine, go to a gym, or use the stairs. Do anything that gets you breathing hard for a while.
- **Keep the horizon close.** "Forever!" is a self-sabotaging idea. The challenge is to not drink for the rest of the day and that is all.
- **Make yourself accountable** by telling other people you are doing this. If you are going to be out alone then arrange a check-in time with them for your expected return.
- **Find and engage in some sort of recovery community** either online or in-person. Other people have done this and can help you, but they can't help if you don't connect to them.
- **Your head is going to tell you lies** to try to get you to drink again, so expect to be lied to. Stopping drinking is necessary, that point is beyond doubt, so don't get into a debate. Recognise the lies as they come and denounce them. You are doing this

because this is what has to happen. There is no argument to be had.

There is a sixteenth thing to do straight-away but its purpose is not to be of immediate help, it is to help later on. I didn't do this and I regretted it bitterly because there were many occasions that I needed this particular piece of evidence to keep me reminded that what I was doing was worth the effort.

- **Write down what it feels like to be you right now.** Find the time as early as possible to record this. This will be important to you later because in a month's time you will not be able to recall this properly; it will be hidden from you. If you are still drinking or have just stopped then describe how you are emotionally and describe what your regular day *feels* like.

A major issue for me early on was that my understanding of the problem was too narrow. I thought the challenge was to stop drinking, but that is not it at all. The challenge is not to stop drinking, but to *stay* stopped. This is a very obvious point but I had somehow missed it completely. If stopping drinking for a spell fixed the problem then that would be the 'treatment' for it. But it isn't, and it isn't because it doesn't work.

If at the height of my drinking I had been put somewhere nice and comfortable, fed, rested and set out in the sunshine every now and again, then I would have got healthy again but I would not have 'recovered' in any enduring sense. As soon as I was let out then I would have gone and got drunk at the earliest opportunity. Stopping drinking does not cure alcoholism. It stops me from being a drunk but that is all. It does nothing to change *why* I drank. That remains and it constantly steers me back towards alcohol. Only when I understood *why* I drank was I able to do the things that would effectively counter-act it. But I had been looking in all the wrong places. I thought I was drinking in response to all the difficulties in my life, "if you understood my problems then you'd drink too", but that was only the surface expression of the problem. The reasons I drank are deeper than this and they are to do with how my brain works in response to alcohol. My mind conspires against my efforts to stop drinking in five distinct ways. The urge to drink (cravings) motivates me to seek out and consume alcohol, the state of my resolve determines my ability to resist this, self-sabotaging thoughts tell me that drinking is a good idea, my memory tells me that drinking was a good experience, and my emotions tell me to drink because that will make me feel better.

All of these conspire to make me drink again but none of these is deliberate or wilful... they all happen entirely automatically. I didn't drink because I made poor choices; I drank because my mind directed me to. As I learned more I started to see the multiple ways that my mind kept turning me towards alcohol. This showed me what I needed to push back against and what actions would do that successfully. Understanding the problem allowed me to distinguish solutions from distractions, but there was also something far more powerful to be won from this.

I needed to stop drinking, and I needed to stay stopped. But I was starting from a position of hopelessness, that is, I was without hope. I had given up trying to give up. I had nothing to grasp hold of because everything I had tried so far had failed. But hope isn't something that magically appears out of nowhere; it has two components that we can deliberately acquire. The first is the belief that the future can be better, and the second is believing that there is a way to get there. I first needed to believe that escape was possible, and then I needed to know how it could be achieved. When I found these then everything turned on a sixpence. The impossible became possible, the path became self-evident, and hope was restored.

Necessary, Possible, and Worthwhile

I didn't stop drinking because I wanted to; I stopped because I had to. If I could have carried on drinking without all the bad things happening then I would have, but this wasn't the case. If I could keep how much I drank to within reasonable limits then I wouldn't have had to stop either, but this too wasn't the case. Perhaps there was a time when this was possible but that time had long since passed. I learned through bitter experience that no matter how hard I tried I could not contain my drinking; it was beyond my means to do so. It could not be done and the proof of this point lay in the simplest and most obvious observation of myself. If I could control my drinking then I would have done so a long time ago. But not only could I not control how much or how often I drank there was another alarming factor; it was getting worse.

The amount that I drank crept up incredibly slowly and it happened so slowly that I didn't notice it. This is one of the immoveable truths about addiction: it is progressive. It always gets worse, never better. Beyond that is an even more disturbing truth: that I never will have control of my drinking. Nobody that has drunk alcoholically has ever gone on to drink normally. Of all of the millions that have attempted this there has not been a single case of an alcoholic going on to become a normal drinker, not one! If the demand to drink outstrips our control then this remains the case forever. The research reveals that I cannot moderate my drinking because the mechanism that does this only works very weakly in me. But not only is this control essentially absent it will remain absent. It is like being born without a limb: we never grow a new one. I can never safely drink again, and the deeper truth is that I never could in the first place.

This was extremely unwelcome news. I could not imagine a life without alcohol. What do people *do* that don't drink? But the idea that all fun in life came through drinking is a lie that my mind created. If drinking was so much fun then how come I ended up so desperate for it to stop? My hopelessly rosy recall of drinking is false, but false or not there is an unavoidable reality: I cannot and never will be able to drink moderately. It will always be excessive and damaging. This truth hurt but it also simplified my options. Whereas I once thought that there were three choices; to carry on drinking as I was, drink sensibly, or (heaven forbid!) stop drinking altogether, I now saw that the middle path was unavailable to me because drinking moderately could never happen. This left me only two options; I could either carry on drinking and my life would continue to get worse and worse, or, and this was the unthinkable thought, I could stop drinking altogether.

While it was obvious to me that the amount I drank had slowly increased over time there were other changes that that I hadn't particularly noticed or that I didn't link to my drinking. What I didn't recognise until it was pointed out to me was that I had slowly changed emotionally. Frequent and heavy drinking changes our underlying mood. It made me feel anxious, unhappy, unsociable, frustrated, with a sense of impending doom, and a racing mind. This mood shift is a direct and inevitable consequence of drinking significantly over an extended period. But these changes didn't just make me feel low; they accelerated the progression of my condition. Alcohol slows our brain down. This makes it less agitated and that makes us calmer. It also makes us more sociable and happier. Alcohol eased distress and cheered me up, and my brain recognised this. So if I was feeling stressed, unhappy or lonely then I was urged to drink, and I made powerful drinking triggers for these emotions. But this is a terrible trap.

I did not know that my lowered emotional state was caused by alcohol, in fact I assumed the very opposite. I thought I was drinking *because* of my stress, anxiety, fear and alone-ness. But the more I drank the worse these got. Alcohol appeared to be the solution to my problems, but that wasn't true; it made them worse.

Alcoholism is progressive and it is progressive in all respects. Yes, the problems it caused in my daily life become more severe but so too did the emotional consequences. I suffered an intensifying descent into hopelessness and despair and this was further fuelled by the burden of shame, guilt and remorse from all the terrible things I had done. If I did nothing to arrest this decline then it would kill me. This may seem like an overdramatic statement but it is not: unchecked alcoholism is fatal. Alcoholics mostly die from; organ failure (liver, kidney, heart, and brain), traumatic injury (vehicle accidents, homicide, accidental injury, or drowning), or, and this is far more common than is acknowledged, suicide.

Stopping drinking was not just something that was desirable, it was essential, because if I did not stop drinking then it would kill me. Continued drinking was ultimately unsurvivable. But knowing that stopping drinking was *necessary* wasn't sufficient in itself to motivate me to stop; I also needed to also believe that it was *worthwhile* and that it was *possible*. It didn't matter how necessary it was that I stopped if I didn't also believe these other two things, because while I didn't believe that it was possible or that it was worthwhile then I wouldn't even bother to try. But neither of these two things was immediately obvious to me. I might have reached the conclusion that stopping drinking had become necessary from my own self-observation, but the evidence proving that it was worthwhile or even possible was less apparent.

One of the great barriers to stopping drinking was that I couldn't imagine a life without alcohol. My experience was that it was the highlight of my day; it was the fun part, the time that I escaped from all my troubles. As my condition progressed, and as I ignored all activities that didn't involve drinking, then alcohol became the *only* fun I could see in my life and the times that I didn't drink were filled with stress, apartness, and anxiety. From this position it appeared that stopping drinking meant forgoing all fun in my life, leaving me with only its hardships, and that was a big call. Who would willingly choose this option? But this perception was entirely incorrect and it was wrong in two ways.

The first is that my drinking had *caused* a lowered emotional state and if I stopped drinking then this depression would correct itself. Stopping drinking doesn't leave us in a permanently miserable state because when we stop drinking then the measures that our brain takes to ward off the effects of alcohol are no longer needed and they are reversed. Drinking stole the means to enjoy myself when I was sober, but when I stopped drinking then that capacity was restored. As the days since my last drink increased then my mood lifted, anxiety faded, and my racing mind calmed down. My mood improved dramatically after I stopped drinking, but while I was still drinking I had no idea that this would happen.

The second falsehood is that my memory is not faithful when it comes to alcohol. My memory associates alcohol with good times and fun but it overlooks all the bad things that come with it. Bad things happened when I drank but these were neither strongly remembered nor were they strongly linked to alcohol. My memory highlighted the good things about drinking and simultaneously minimised the bad things. But those bad things were really, really, serious! This failure to see the whole picture, to only see the upsides, gave me an impossibly favourable view of alcohol. I have a recall of drinking that is incorrectly positive and from this position it looked like if I stopped drinking then I would be losing all fun in my life. But the truth is that my drinking was far less fun than I remember and the damage that it caused was far, far worse. When I stopped drinking then all the bad stuff would stop too, but my mind didn't rush to point this out to me. It wasn't at all obvious to me as I set out, in fact I anticipated the opposite, but stopping drinking was enormously uplifting. Stopping drinking dramatically improved how I felt within myself and about my place in the world. When I stopped drinking then my life got better and this is what *must* happen otherwise nobody would ever succeed. If people went through all the effort and struggle of stopping drinking and they were still miserable then there would be no point in continuing to struggle; they might as well drink again, and they would. But people that have stopped drinking universally say that their lives got better, and despite what I expected I was not miserable sober. When I stopped drinking my mood lifted, my anxiety faded, my racing mind calmed down, hopelessness disappeared, and my capacity to find joy was restored.

For me to be able to stop drinking I had to believe that it was necessary, that it was worthwhile, and also that it was possible. If I did not believe it was possible to stop then all I was achieving by trying to do so was to delay when I would have my next drink. If that was the case then I might as well end the struggle and drink again now. I cannot sustain the effort required to stop drinking if I do not believe that it is possible. But my experience in this regard was not promising. If you have taken the trouble to pick up this book then this will not be the first time you have tried to do something about your drinking. You will have already tried numerous times and those attempts will have failed every time. We all experience this. Whether these were attempts to limit the amount we drank, how often we drank, or when, where or what we permitted ourselves to drink, they all failed. We tried to limit our drinking to certain days and occasions, and we tried to stop for specific periods, but we couldn't keep it going and always ended up drinking exactly like we did before. My experience of stopping drinking was not promising, in fact my experience was that it was not possible, and if it was not possible to stop drinking then why would I waste the time and effort trying?

Just like my memory created the illusion that stopping drinking was not worthwhile it also supported the illusion that it was not possible. But this was incorrect. This was only true for *my* efforts, and it was only true for those efforts to date. It is most certainly not true for the millions that have successfully done it. It isn't easy but I didn't need some extraordinary super-power to be able to stop drinking, what I needed was to realise that it was possible and that it was possible for me, and I didn't find that realisation by looking inwards. The best proof that stopping drinking is possible is to be found in those that have done it, and those people are easy enough to find. People that have stopped drinking can be met in any community based recovery group and they can be found in online communities and they all say the same thing. They say it is hard to do, but that it is incredibly worthwhile.

I needed help because I had tried everything I could think of and everything had failed, so I walked into a recovery meeting hoping to find something that would work. In truth I was hoping to find ways to manage my drinking and keep it under control, but I didn't get that. What I saw was a group of ordinary looking people who were calm and cheerful and who had all done something that I thought was impossible: they had all stopped drinking. It was possible! Up until 1953 it was though that climbing Mount Everest was impossible because all attempts, no matter how well prepared, had failed. But once Hillary and Tensing showed it was possible then suddenly lots of people could do it. People had not suddenly become more capable, and the mountain had not suddenly become less challenging, it was their perception that had changed. I felt a similar change. I left that meeting with something I hadn't had in years: hope. I had seen that stopping drinking was possible and that it was possible for ordinary folk. This was essential evidence for me and it fundamentally changed my determination, so do the same. Go to a recovery meeting, in person or online, and look for two pieces of evidence: that it is possible to stop drinking, and that it is worthwhile. Everything else that is said or done there is immaterial. What is needed is no more than these two proofs because this knowledge radically changes how we see the problem, and removing those internal barriers makes everything possible.

I didn't choose to become an alcoholic, and I can't choose it to be different. It is what it is, and I had to learn to overcome it if I was to survive. But the success of my effort depended on me being able to hold firm to three core beliefs; that it was necessary to stop drinking, that it was possible to stop drinking, and that the effort required to do so was worthwhile. A failure of any of these beliefs would see me drink again so it was vital that I made them as secure as I possibly could. Seek out the evidence that proves these three things to your complete satisfaction and do whatever it takes to keep yourself reminded of them. Record it in a journal, leave notes on the fridge, or write it on the living room wall if that is what it takes, but these beliefs must remain unshakeable because they are going to be challenged and they are going to be challenged severely.

My mind conspires against me mercilessly. While I had made a decision to stop drinking I had only done so in the conscious, thoughtful part of my brain. But the parts of my brain that are invisible to me and operate automatically still wanted me to drink, and they never get tired. My mind has a limitless capacity to talk me into drinking again so if my recovery is not built on an immoveable foundation then I will bring down my own effort. At first the challenge was enormous and the rewards were small but over time the positions reversed and I reached a place where the effort is small but the gains are huge. What I most needed was the ability to stay the course in order to reap those gains and the three fundamental truths, that stopping drinking is necessary, stopping drinking is possible, and stopping drinking is worthwhile were my back-stop when all else had failed. The test is fierce and relentless at first but these three beliefs carried me through the tough times. They will keep us safe but only if we keep *them* safe, so make them strong. Take the time now to gather and record the proof that these three things are not only true, but that they are true beyond all doubt. The evidence is to be found within you and in those that have recovered, so seek it out and record it.

Stopping drinking is necessary and this isn't even up for debate. Record the worst things that have happened because of your drinking and record how they made you feel. Now factor-in that alcoholism is progressive. While we continue to drink then things continue to get worse. What is the next step on that descent, and the next, and where does it end up?

Stopping drinking is possible and worthwhile, but you don't know that for sure yet, so go to the people that do. We can read peoples' recovery stories in books but hearing it first-hand is far more persuasive, so find that. Engage in a recovery program, online or in person. Do this even if your only reason to do so is to get answers to these questions. "Is it possible?" and "is it worthwhile?". Directly ask the people there for their experience: what was it like and what is it like now? They were once in your position and will understand exactly why you need to know this. They will help if you ask because the sole purpose of these groups is to help each other. If you never engage in the group again but get answers to these questions then it will still be well worth that one visit.

These three beliefs are the rampart we stand behind when we fight, so they need to be unbreachable. Do everything you can to shore up these defences because they *will* be tested. A war is coming; a war with your own mind.

Cravings and Triggers

Addiction is not simply a habit, it is habit enforced by chemical compulsion. My brain has about 85 billion neurons (brain cells) in it and each of these connects to about 7,000 others. Signals are passed between them and they operate in linked bunches to form to a single idea or action. When the same bundle of neurons gets activated regularly then their action gets stronger and faster and this bunch becomes a quicker path through my brain: it reaches a conclusion earlier than other paths; it comes up with an answer first. This is what a habit is. In many circumstances I may find that "have a drink" is the first thought to arrive, but if it was only an idea that arrived before the others then I wouldn't feel the need to act on it, I could choose from my options. What is different about this idea is that when it arrives it comes with added compulsion in the form of a chemical called dopamine. Dopamine is what causes the compelling "wanting" or "longing for" sensation of a craving.

There was one thing about my drinking that I couldn't understand at all. I was perfectly capable in every other aspect of my life but for some bizarre reason I could not control my drinking. I drank more than I wanted to, I drank more often than I wanted to, I drank at times and on occasions that I shouldn't, and I couldn't stop any of it. This inability to control my drinking when everybody else could was beyond confusing. It seemed like I didn't have an "off" switch when it came to alcohol, and it turns out that this is literally the case.

I get the very clear sensation that alcohol draws me towards it but this is not what is happening at all because there is no mechanism by which alcohol can exert such a force over me. The mechanism works the other way around. Alcohol does not pull *me* towards *it*, *I* am being pushed towards *alcohol*, but I don't recognise this because the push comes from a part of my mind that I can't see into.

When an urge to drink comes on me it doesn't come because I've somehow willed it to, it comes entirely automatically, and there is no conscious thinking involved whatsoever. Sometimes I get a gentle longing for a drink, sometimes I get the idea that a drink would be really good, and sometimes I get the flat-out, primal scream: "I need a drink now!" These are all cravings and they are all caused by the same mental mechanism. The only thing that differs is their intensity. Cravings may vary in intensity but they don't come randomly. They are "triggered" into existence by parts of my brain that are collectively known as the "dopamine reward system".

The reward system is a group of connected parts that work together to encourage me to do things that aid my survival and to discourage me from doing things that could be dangerous or harmful. It is located in the subconscious part of my brain which means it is invisible to me and I have no knowledge whatsoever of what it is doing. I am no more aware of the operations of the reward system than I am of the processes that regulate my breathing or heartbeat, but its action is what propels addiction. My memory tells me "what it is" and the reward system tells me "what to do", then it urges me to take that action. But it doesn't encourage me to act in a particular way with words or ideas; it releases a chemical in my brain that motivates me to act. That chemical is called dopamine and its compelling power is not to be underestimated: it is what makes me pick up that next drink even though I know for certain it will give me a hangover.

The reward system works by motivating me to do the things that I have discovered to be good for me and by discouraging me from repeating the things that I have been found to be bad. It evolved well before humans did, all animals have it, and it was a huge evolutionary advance over instinct. There is no way to predict all the things that might help or harm me throughout my lifetime, I meet new ones as I go along, and the reward system is self-learning. As I encounter more things that are good for me or bad for me then the successful behaviour for each circumstance is remembered; approach or move away. The next time I meet that circumstance then I am urged by a release of dopamine to repeat the action that was successful before. When I begin that action then the dopamine release is immediately stopped, the nagging urge that encouraged me to act is removed, and I feel an immediate sense of relief. The "aaahhh!" sense of ease and comfort that I get on taking my first drink is not caused by alcohol. It can't be caused by the alcohol because I get the sensation of relief *before* the alcohol has had time to enter my bloodstream and be carried to my brain. The sense of ease and comfort that I get on taking our first drink is created by the reward system. It is the relief I get when the nagging of dopamine, urging me to drink, is suddenly stopped.

In alcoholics the reward system latches onto alcohol as something very beneficial and it urges me to drink whenever alcohol is available or nearby. It remembers the circumstances that have yielded alcohol before and it forms a new association of a circumstance (like a particular bar for example) and an action (have a drink!) for each of them. We call these "drinking triggers" and each time I drink in a new circumstance then a new trigger is formed. But the reward system doesn't just make triggers; it reinforces existing ones if they are successful. If I am encouraged to seek alcohol by a trigger and then do so then this trigger was a successful one. Triggers that deliver the outcome sought are more valuable than the ones that fail and the reward system deliberately strengthens the successful ones. If a drinking trigger is successful in securing alcohol then its power is raised by increasing the amount of dopamine that it releases, and this makes the motivating urge that it launches more intense. The next craving that this trigger launches will be more powerful. This is why the compulsion to drink steadily increases over time.

Evolution made the reward system impart urgency to doing things that benefit my survival. However, something beneficial, like a food that is available right now, might not be found again for some time so the reward system encourages me to take advantage of the opportunity while it is present; but it also encourages me to do so efficiently. If for example there is a bird in the middle of a field of fruiting berry bushes then there are berries all around it. There is good food in every direction but it would be inefficient in terms of energy use for the bird to randomly pick berries from all corners of the field. So the reward system evolved to use energy efficiently by encouraging the bird to take the closest fruit first. The motivating urge launched by a trigger is stronger when its subject is closer than when the subject is more distant, and in terms of alcohol this means that a craving to drink is far more powerful when I am close to the circumstances of a drinking trigger than it is when I am some distance from it. This knowledge becomes useful when we come to stopping drinking.

For me this means that if I begin drinking in a location where alcohol is freely available then I am close to many triggers. I can see alcohol, I can smell alcohol, I can see people drinking, I can hear the noises of drinking and so on; I am surrounded by triggers. This means that I will experience a new craving for a drink as soon as I have finished the one in front of me and this craving will be powerful because the triggering circumstances are close. This property of triggers is why, when I walked into a bar or other venue where alcohol was available, then I ended up drinking more and drinking for longer than I intended to when I first stepped in.

Every new circumstance in which I drink forms a new trigger and my brain constantly scans incoming information looking for trigger circumstances that have been met before. Directly seeing or smelling alcohol will make those particular triggers fire, but triggers are by no means limited to this direct identification. I make drinking triggers for places at which I've drunk previously but I also make triggers for things that are more abstract. I routinely drank; with certain people, to certain music, at certain types of event, at certain times of the day, and on certain days of the week, and I made drinking triggers for all of these. Over time I accumulated hundreds and hundreds of triggers and they each encouraged me to drink whenever they were fired. The cravings brought on by these triggers grew stronger each time I acted on them and they grew stronger as I drew closer to the trigger's location. But the reward system can be misled when it comes to closeness.

The reward system evolved before our human ability to visualise and imagine and it evolved independently of them; they aren't directly connected. It also evolved long before the existence of pictures, photographs, and television etc. and while my conscious mind (the part I can see into) knows that these aren't real my subconscious mind (the part I can't see into) does not.

My subconscious mind can't tell the difference between a glass containing alcohol and a picture of a glass containing alcohol: it recognises both of these as though they are real. This means that seeing a picture of alcohol or even imagining it will cause a trigger to fire. I can bring powerful cravings on myself by simply thinking about drinking and this causes problems when I try to stop. But regardless of how they are triggered, or how intense they are, all cravings are have one thing in common: they are all time-limited.

When a bird is in the vicinity of a bush that it has fed at successfully before then dopamine is released to make it want to go there again: it gets a craving. But what if that bush has been stripped of its fruit? If the reward system only motivated the bird to go there, and continued that motivation until the bird fed, then the bird would be urged to stay there forever for no benefit. It would waste effort and it would waste time. But the reward system improved over millions of years to use limited energy resources both effectively and efficiently. So the bird does not sit there waiting forever because this would be neither efficient nor effective. If the bird finds food at the bush then it continues to be motivated to stay and feed and the triggers that directed it there are strengthened. But if there isn't any food there then the trigger stops releasing dopamine after a while and the motivating urge stops. When this happens then the bird is no longer motivated towards that particular bush and it moves on to look for food elsewhere. My cravings to drink do exactly the same thing. If a trigger is fired then I am urged to drink. But if no alcohol is forthcoming in response to that urge then the trigger gives up and the craving ceases after a few minutes. This is another really important thing to know when it comes to stopping drinking: cravings are time-limited.

The intensity of a craving is determined by how close I am to the circumstances of its trigger and by the number of times that this trigger has been successful in delivering alcohol. The triggers of the reward system steadily encouraged me to drink more and they encouraged me to drink more often, and my drinking triggers strengthened without limit. They also increased in number and I ended up being triggered to drink by almost everything, almost everywhere, and almost all of the time. But everybody has this reward system, so how come that everyone that ever has a drink doesn't become an alcoholic?

The reward system evolved to encourage some behaviour and to discourage others, but a single subject can have multiple triggers for different circumstances. For example, I have two triggers for lemons. I may feel the urge to squeeze some lemon juice over fried food, but I would recoil strongly from the suggestion that I should eat a whole one. That recoil, the urge to move away, comes straight from the reward system. Just like the example of the lemon most people have some triggers that encourage them to drink alcohol and other triggers that urge them not to. Wait! What? People have triggers that urge them to *not* drink? Yes they do, but we don't. Normal drinkers have triggers motivating against drinking too much and they have triggers motivating against drinking at the wrong times. They have triggers linked to the discomforts of drinking too much like hangovers, vomiting, and loss of control, and they have triggers relating to the unwanted consequences of drinking; failing to meet important obligations, doing things that are regretted or shameful and so on. But alcohol-avoiding triggers do not form well in me. The reward system of a normal drinker learns from their bad drinking experiences and it forms alcohol-avoiding triggers to deter them from repeating these mistakes. But I don't form these triggers well and I don't learn from my mistakes when it comes to alcohol. It isn't that my reward system lacks the means to form them, the error is that they are not recognised as actions to be avoided, and it is this error that makes me susceptible to addiction.

People are not identical. There is enormous variability in our physical appearance, there is enormous variability within our brains, and this variability extends into the reward system. My reward system encourages me to proceed with or to avoid certain actions based on whether they've been helpful or harmful to me in the past. But it is how the reward system decides which is which that is crucial to addiction. One of the defining behaviours of alcoholics is that we continue to drink despite that drinking having repeated, adverse outcomes. But this is precisely what the reward system is supposed to prevent from happening. The reward system is supposed to *discourage* us from repeating experiences that were found to be harmful. So what is happening here?

The reward system sits in my subconscious mind and is made up of several parts; one of these is the amygdala. The brain has two memory systems, the hippocampus and the amygdala. The hippocampus remembers plain information; details, incidents, and facts, and the amygdala remembers emotions related to those details. It is the hippocampus that allows me to recognise my cousin, and it is my amygdala that tells me that I like him. But the amygdala is part of a connected system that directs behaviour. It determines if something is good or bad and then it either activates a trigger or forms a new one. If a new occurrence is a good one then it creates an encouraging trigger and if it is a bad one then it creates an aversive trigger... and this is where my brain makes a terrible mistake when it comes to alcohol.

My reward system uses the amygdala to decide what things are good and what things are bad, but it isn't always obvious which is which. Consider these two examples.

- There is some good fruit high in a tree. I can climb the tree and take the fruit, but there is a risk that I might fall and injure myself. Which is the better action, boldness or caution?
- If there is a bush bearing ripening fruit then I can either take a little barely-ripe fruit now or come back tomorrow when there will be more that has ripened. But if I leave it until tomorrow then someone else may have come and taken the fruit before me. Which is the better option, act now or later?

There are advantages and disadvantages to each action and there is no clear or reliable best choice, but the amygdala *always* makes a choice because indecision in the wild can be fatal. Which conclusion it will reach depends on whether the reward is worth more than the cost (e.g. the effort, the pain, the discomfort, or the time), and which choice we make varies from person to person. If it did not then we would all react in precisely the same way in any given circumstance. But there is significant variation across the population. I discount risk quite strongly and would climb the tree to get the fruit. I also discount delay quite strongly and would take the fruit now rather than later. It turns out that these are the internal preferences that favour addiction.

Someone whose amygdala recognises risk more strongly than I do, and who recognises "later" as being more important than me, will form completely different triggers when it comes to alcohol. Their amygdala recognises the penalties that come with drinking more strongly than I do so their reward system will form triggers discouraging it when mine will not. Also, many of the consequences of drinking occur much later than at the time that I drink, so their reward system recognises these and forms triggers against them, but again, mine does not. It is the thresholds at which my amygdala determines what activity is risky, and what later consequences are considered relevant, that dictate whether it will form an alcohol-avoiding trigger or an alcohol-seeking trigger. *My* threshold settings guarantee that I will almost always make drinking triggers and only rarely make alcohol-avoiding ones. These two deep characteristics; favouring the prize more strongly than the potential penalty, and favouring something now rather than something later, serve me perfectly well in every other aspect of my life, but when it comes to drinking they serve me terribly because my reward system gets alcohol wrong. Alcohol became bad for me, and I should have been motivated away from it, but my reward system failed to recognise this.

Now here is the stinger. I did not "learn" these internal settings, they are predetermined like instinct, and I was born with them. Current research shows that the internal values that my amygdala uses for decision-making are genetically prescribed. If my parents carry the genes that set these thresholds unhelpfully then it is perfectly likely that I will inherit them. But they can equally well occur within the range of normal variability.

I value the prize more than the penalty, and I prefer something now far more strongly than something later. The combined effect of these two internal preferences is that I make many alcohol-seeking triggers but very few alcohol-avoiding triggers. I am more often directed towards alcohol than I am away from it and the more often I drink then the more I strengthen those triggers. My reward system encourages me to drink more and the act of drinking further strengthens the triggers to do so. This is a self-reinforcing loop which once begun puts my reward system into a runaway state whereby the desire to drink becomes increasingly more compelling, and there is no upper limit to this. But we are not all equally susceptible to addiction. Whether I build alcohol-seeking triggers or alcohol-avoiding triggers depends on the internal settings that my reward system uses, and the thresholds for these vary between individuals. Susceptibility to addiction isn't on or off, it depends how strongly we discount risk and how strongly we discount delay and each of these is themselves a variable. In round terms there is about 15% of the population that is susceptible to addiction and some people are more susceptible than others. But 85% of the population is never at risk of alcoholism because their alcohol-avoiding triggers prevent it. People that are highly susceptible only need a tiny push to tip their reward system into a runaway condition, and for many their first drink is sufficient. Those that are slightly less susceptible may need to drink frequently for a sustained period, strengthening their alcohol-seeking triggers, before their reward system enters this runaway state. But susceptibility to addiction is not the same as predestination. Even if I *am* susceptible to addiction then I could carry this vulnerability through my whole life and be unaffected by it if I never drank or if I never drank sufficiently to tip my reward system into this self-reinforcing condition. I am not blameless, but I *was* unaware.

People that are highly susceptible to addiction do not need to drink often before the power of their drinking triggers commits their trajectory, and many report becoming hooked from their first experience. Many that drank from their early teens say that alcohol set them free socially, but it didn't last. They drank in exactly the same way as their friends did but they ended up trapped and isolated by alcohol and their friends didn't. They were in the 15% and their friends were in the 85% but they had no way of knowing this. There is a high prevalence of alcoholism among people that drank heavily in their youth but this isn't because youth drinking is a causal factor in addiction; it is that this is most likely our first encounter with alcohol and it will activate addiction in the more susceptible. Most people that drink significantly in their youth will *not* go on to become alcoholic, but many of the 15% do.

Alcoholism is not randomly distributed across the population; it is more prominent in some societal settings than others. But this isn't because those circumstances cause addiction; it is because these circumstances are likely to activate the susceptibility where it is present. If people are raised in heavy-drinking households or are actively engaged in heavy-drinking social circles then they are likely to activate that susceptibility where it exists. Also people that drink for relief from some distress in their life; work stress, family stress, prolonged hardship etc. will very likely activate any susceptibility, and if people drink for relief from the persistent trauma of some abuse then they will almost certainly set addiction in motion if that susceptibility exists in them.

None of these circumstances directly *causes* addiction, what they do is they dramatically increase the likelihood that the susceptibility, where it exists, will become activated. Each of these circumstances leads people to drink repeatedly and it is *this* that activates addiction in those that are susceptible to it. This why the prevalence of addiction is strongly clustered around these societal groups, and what they have in common is that they all encourage frequent drinking.

But even if we don't fall into one of these categories then the chance that anyone who is significantly susceptible to addiction will avoid it in our contemporary western society is remarkably small. Drinking compulsively is very heavily frowned upon but drinking itself is not, in fact society expects that we *will* drink. If we did not drink frequently for any other reason then we would drink to conform to societal norms and this in itself could be enough to engage susceptibility where it exists and commit our decline.

I had the vague awareness that I seemed to have no "off" switch when it came to alcohol but I didn't realise that this is quite literally true. Normal drinkers are urged away from alcohol if it isn't an appropriate time or place to drink and they are urged away from alcohol when having more is a bad idea, but I am not, I am still urged towards it. It is not that I make bad choices when it comes to drinking it is that the normal means to make good ones is absent in me. I have no "off" switch. Mine is permanently fixed in the "on" position and this set me on a course with catastrophic consequences. I didn't get to be this way because I applied poor control and drank too much. I got to be this way because I was born with two perfectly common internal characteristics that combined have disastrous implications. Other people are sometimes motivated away from alcohol and this prevents over-strengthening of their drinking triggers, but I am only ever encouraged to drink and never to slow down or desist. The absence of these alcohol-avoiding triggers means that my condition is progressive: it *always* becomes more severe, and it will *never* get better on its own. I can never bring my drinking under control because the mechanism to apply that control is absent in me.

The triggers of my reward system are unbalanced when it comes to alcohol, and they always will be. The option to carry on drinking, but to do so moderately, does not and never will exist for me because I am, and always will be, motivated to drink more strongly than I am motivated against it. Stopping for a spell does not change this. I can never drink moderately, and my only survivable course is to stop completely.

Once I understood how cravings and triggers worked then I could use this knowledge to help myself stop drinking, but there was one more really important thing to know about them. The triggers of the reward system, once established, remain in place forever. This is a general feature of how the brain works: what has become known cannot become unknown. Once a trigger has been formed then it can never be removed and neither can its associated motivating urge. But while a trigger can never be removed the strength of the motivating urge that it invokes *can* be changed... and this is our way out.

The reward system aids survival but in the wild the availability of something beneficial like an important food can be unpredictable and the reward system accommodates this variability. For example, if a bird learns to visit a bush because it gives good fruit then the reward system motivates it to return to the bush and look for more food. But if the bush stops producing fruit altogether, like at the end of its season, then the reward system will bring an unwanted result. If the motivating urge continues then the bird will still keep visiting it forever for no gain. This is an inefficient use of the bird's resources so the reward system evolved to accommodate this circumstance. Firstly, the cravings that are invoked have a limited time-span. If there isn't any fruit available at the bush when the bird visits then the urge to continue to search there fades after several minutes and it loses interest and moves on. But importantly, if things stop happening the way that a trigger anticipates, then the importance of that trigger is lowered. In exactly the same way that a trigger is strengthened by repeated success it is weakened by repeated failure. When a trigger consistently fails to return the outcome sought then the importance of acting on it (the intensity of the craving it launches) is reduced. My brain can't unlearn that alcohol has been identified as something to be sought out, but the importance of securing it *can* be changed, and it is by not drinking in response to cravings that I reduce their intensity.

By successively *not* drinking in response to cravings my reward system recognises that the likelihood of the drinking triggers being successful is less than anticipated, and the urgency given to finding alcohol is progressively reduced. This is an incredibly important piece of information for anyone attempting to stop drinking:

Every time I resist a craving then the intensity of the next craving launched by its trigger is diminished.

I didn't start out being addicted; I started out drinking like everyone else. But when my triggers strengthened and my drinking became compulsive then society suddenly determined that I was bad, weak and immoral. But people reached this conclusion based on their own experience. They assume that I get the same prompting away from alcohol that they do but ignore it, and this is why they condemn my behaviour. They do not know that I get no such motivation away from alcohol. Nor do they know that I am only ever motivated to seek it and to seek it now. They assume that I make poor choices whereas in fact I am never given any choice to make. In me the decision to drink is already made and it is made automatically and invisibly. People make judgements about alcoholics based on incorrect assumptions and the shame they cast is undeserved, but I learned to forgive them for that because they have no need to know any better. But I do need to know because once I understand how addiction behaves in me then I can anticipate its moves and directly counter them instead of flailing around and randomly stabbing in the dark.

All my problems with alcohol start with the reward system and compound out from there. But I can make the demands of the reward system diminish in intensity by overcoming the cravings it produces, and this is the essential focus of our early efforts. I did not manage to stop drinking because I got better at resisting the cravings, though I did get better at navigating them. I became able to stop drinking by successively denying cravings, because when I did this then their intensity gradually fell to a level that I could step past them without them disturbing my daily life. It took enormous effort to do this but slowly the compulsion to drink faded into the background, and this is the pathway out of addiction.

Managing Cravings

Whether or not I will drink at any moment boils down to an incredibly simple equation: - If the urge to drink exceeds the will to resist it then I will drink. There are two components here: - the intensity of the desire to drink, and the determination to overcome it.

Overcoming cravings is exhausting and it places me at risk because wears down my resolve. My mind's ability to demand that I drink is limitless whereas my determination to fend it off is finite, but neither of these two is entirely fixed. This piece knowledge is enormously helpful because it shows us that we can tackle the problem from both ends: cravings *and* resolve. There are things I can do that will lessen the impact of the cravings, and there are things I can do that will preserve my resolve. So the plan for the first few hours, days and weeks is twofold: - do the things that reduce the call to drink, and also do the things that increase resolve. This dramatically reduces the chances of experiencing a powerful craving at a time when resolve is insufficient to overcome it. It also lifts the chances of success because knowing *how* a task is to be achieved greatly increases my belief that I can complete it. Having a plan gave focus to what I did and allowed me to keep my efforts on track. When I found myself struggling then I could look at what I was doing and compare it to the plan. Was I doing all of the things that I should? Had I stopped doing something that I should be doing? Or had I started doing something that I shouldn't?

This chapter looks at the things that can be done to reduce the intensity of that demand to drink, but before that there is a particular circumstance that everyone in recovery will meet and there are some specific things that can be done to address the challenges that it poses. I met the fiercest cravings I ever encountered during withdrawal. But I didn't have to simply grit my teeth and push through it; there were things I could do to make my path easier.

Withdrawal:

The symptoms of withdrawal are not caused by the absence of alcohol but by the presence of chemicals released into my brain and body to ward off its effects. When I abruptly stop drinking then alcohol no longer nullifies their potency and I feel them fully for the first time. The principal effect of alcohol on the brain is that it slows everything down and when I drank frequently and heavily then my brain speeded things up in several ways to try to counter this. When I drank frequently then my brain not only reacted to the presence of alcohol it *anticipated* that it was going to be slowed down by alcohol and it speeded everything up in preparation for this. I didn't normally feel the full effects of these changes because I would drink again and this counteracted their effect. But when I abruptly stopped drinking then for the first time I could feel the full impact of what my body did every day to try to keep me functional while I drank: - I had a central nervous system that was hugely over-excited and a highly elevated heart rate. The over-excitement of my central nervous system produced 'the shakes', a racing mind, and anxiety, and the elevated heart activity gave me a thumping heart and high blood pressure. Usually these symptoms would be removed by drinking but when I stopped completely then this no longer happened. The chemicals that increased my heart and brain function were released at a rate my brain considered optimal for the conditions that existed while I drank and these chemicals were *still* released at that same rate once I stopped. But the effects of these chemicals accumulated once there was no daily dose of alcohol cancelling their effect. This is why the symptoms of withdrawal get worse for two or three days before gradually receding. It took my brain a while to recognise that the measures it was taking in anticipation of alcohol were now harmful rather than helpful, so the effects of withdrawal increased in severity until that happened. But once my brain recognised that the defensive measures it took against a daily assault of alcohol were causing more harm than good then it started to step them down and the impacts of withdrawal subsided.

The symptoms of withdrawal are mostly caused by the over excitement of the heart and nervous system by the neurotransmitters and hormones that kept me safe, alert, and functional while I drank. How severely we will be affected by these depends on our personal physiology and also how aggressively our body has been defending itself against the sedative effect of alcohol. Some people will only be mildly affected but some will struggle with heart irregularities and confusion, even hallucinations, but one thing is certain. If I have drunk enough, and I have drunk often enough, for me to need to stop drinking altogether then I am definitely going to experience *some* uncomfortable consequences when that alcohol is abruptly absent. My heart pounded, our mind raced, and my anxiety went through the roof. All of these symptoms would be eased if I would only have a drink and my mind screamed out for alcohol. The cravings I encountered during withdrawal were the most intense I ever experienced and at times they were virtually continuous. I clearly remember being on my knees in my bedroom, face buried in a pillow crying, and screaming for it to stop. This is why the most likely time to give up and drink again is within the first week of stopping, and it isn't a little more likely, it is *by far* the most likely. But withdrawal is entirely predictable for anyone that has drunk over an extended period. It is definitely coming and it is going to bring on intense and non-stop cravings. So if the plan is to succeed by reducing the impact cravings have on us then this is the place start.

Medical science does not leave us entirely to our own devices when it comes to withdrawal and cravings; there are things that can be done. A doctor can advise on whether or not supervision through withdrawal is prudent and they can also prescribe medication that will reduce brain and heart stimulation through this period. This will reduce the risk of severe health consequences as well as reducing anxiety and the severity of cravings. I did not seek advice and that was a mistake. Looking back I can't tell if it was ignorance or pride that prevented me from getting help but I should have because it would have avoided unnecessary struggle and hardship. I know I was at least vaguely aware that help through withdrawal was available so I can only assume that pride was the barrier. I didn't want to admit my problem to my doctor for fear of being judged, but that was foolishness because doctors see this every day. I should have taken the help that was available and this was a mistake I can see clearly with hindsight.

At first it was the cravings that were the biggest challenge to me stopping drinking, but this wasn't only difficult through withdrawal it was ongoing. It took months for the cravings to subside to a level that I could casually brush them aside and throughout that time I had to get past them without drinking. I had to do this every single time because if the strength of a craving *ever* exceeded my will to resist it then I would drink again. There were ways to help myself with this: - I could reduce the number of cravings I experienced, I could reduce the intensity and duration of those cravings, and I could reduce the occasions when one craving subsided only to be replaced by another. Finally, I could learn ways to successfully navigate the cravings that I *did* experience.

Reducing the number of cravings:

The aim was to reduce the severity of cravings to the point that I could walk past them without breaking my stride. We reduce the power of the drinking triggers that launch cravings by successively experiencing cravings but not drinking in response to them. When we do this then our brain actively steps down the power of the trigger (and therefore lowers the intensity of the craving it launches). Cravings don't just fade away on their own when we stop drinking. The power of an established trigger is retained in case it becomes useful again one day, so not only is resisting cravings the way to reduce their intensity, it is the *only* way.

I needed to meet and overcome cravings because that is how to make their triggers decline in strength. Ultimately I had to face the cravings of all of my drinking triggers if I was to take the power out of them, but I didn't have to face them all on 'Day One'; I could spread them out. The plan is to lower the impact of cravings to avoid collapsing under the load, and one way of doing this was to remove some triggers from my daily routine. Many of my most powerful triggers were well known to me and I could deliberately take some of these out of my life for a while. I wasn't stopping these triggers from being problematic, I still had to address them at some point, what I was doing was deferring *when* I would deal with them. There were some straightforward things to do that significantly lightened the load for a while: -

I didn't go into the places I used to drink. I didn't go into places that sold alcohol. I wouldn't even pull into the car park of anywhere that sold alcohol. I changed my normal routes so that I didn't drive past the places I used to drink at or the places I used to buy alcohol from and I didn't have alcohol in the house.

I could not expect to be able to get sober if I walked into a bar every day after work because it wasn't going to happen. I could not expect to walk into a liquor store and always come out with only lemonade. I could not expect that I would forever stay out of my favourite watering hole if I went past it every day, and I could not expect to be able to leave alcohol in a bottle if I had some at home; I wouldn't. Keeping a bottle or two in the house so that I could be polite and offer it to a visitor was delusional because the only person that was ever going to drink that was me. I could get away with any of these things some of the time, but if I met the craving they launched at the same time as my resolve was low then they would catch me out; it was only a matter of time. I couldn't trust myself to behave rationally when it came to alcohol and I had learned this through years of bitter experience. If I was going to stop drinking then I needed to move myself away from alcohol for a while. So I avoided all these things until I became confident that I could manage the risk they presented. But the circumstances that triggered the most powerful and persistent cravings were unavoidable, and these were the times at which I routinely drank.

There were patterns to the times at which I drank; evenings, afternoons, lunchtimes, weekends etc. and all of these times were triggering. But of them all it was the time after I left work that was the most difficult. This was a time that I'd routinely drunk for years and as far as my brain was concerned that was what I *should* be doing right then. The problem with this time is that it was chock-full of triggers and I had to make big changes to reduce the number of times that my mind would be screaming at me to drink. I changed the route I took home from work and this avoided going past many of the places that I either drank or bought alcohol at. That was a start but once home I would be confronted by the demand to drink for an extended period. The issue here wasn't that I needed to get past a single craving, it was that I needed to get through a period of time spanning one or two hours during which time the cravings would be almost continuous. I needed to be fully occupied through that period or else my mind would zero in on alcohol and stay there. I painted the house, all of it, inside and out and that worked really well for me. This gave me something to do as soon as I got home. I would spend the journey home planning what I was going to do next and in what order, and once there I had a job to do straight away that commanded my full attention. This meant my mind had little capacity to wander off and dwell on thoughts of drinking. There were days I couldn't raise the enthusiasm to start but I had to force myself past those moments otherwise I was definitely going to struggle against drinking for the next hour or so. At the end of the period I always got a lift from what I'd done because I had achieved something worthwhile and performing that task had carried me through the most difficult part of my day more easily.

I painted the house but there were plenty of other things I could do that would have worked just as well. What I'd needed was something that would last an hour or two, would go on for several weeks (months before I'd really finished), kept my mind and hands fully occupied, and left me with a sense of achievement when I stopped. There are many things I could have done that fitted this description. I could have done something that benefitted my health like some sport or exercise, I could have engaged in some creative venture like music or art, I could have learned something new; a skill, a craft, an educational course of some sort, I could have engaged in some sort of community work that helped others, or I could have embarked on some other major project that I'd always wanted to do but never had the time. I had that time now. I could have spent that time fretting and stressing about not being able to have a drink but I instead used it in such a way that those thoughts never had the opportunity to settle in and grow.

I knew when the most challenging times of the day and week were so there was no excuse for me not doing something to help myself through these periods. There are innumerable ways to deal with these times but the most important thing to do was to find one *and do it*. Activities that made me feel more capable, or more loveable, or more valued, or more worthy, were the best because these not only kept me usefully occupied they also provide a lift in my self-esteem, and that was in desperate need of repair.

However I negotiated these periods the main thing was to fill those times with some sort of deliberate activity because sitting idle at those times was guaranteed bringing on severe cravings. Time alone with my thoughts was always challenging because not only can no-one see me ("no-one will know!") but my racing mind churned and tumbled over all my problems. One bad memory linked in another, then another, and soon my mind was a tangled mess of all my troubles and my mind demanded relief from them.

There is an automatic process of our mind that keeps bringing back unhelpful thoughts and here is a simple illustration of it working. Sometimes in conversation I will struggle to remember a specific detail; someone's name, a product name, a place etc. Then, hours or even days later, when I am a long way from the occasion that required it, the answer suddenly pops into my head. Our mind does this all the time with unresolved information. The brain evolved to keep information organised, unambiguous and orderly. It doesn't like unsatisfactory or unresolved information because that can lead to indecision, and this could be fatal in the wild. So the things that it doesn't like continue to be worked on to try to bring them to a satisfactory conclusion whenever our brain has some idle-time. This happens in our subconscious mind (the part we *can't* see into) but will cross into our conscious mind (the part we *can* see into) whenever there is processing capacity available. This is why time alone is so difficult, because this is the time that all the unsatisfactory things, past and present, come charging into our consciousness in search of resolution. For as long as I am thinking about these issues, whether it is in the conscious part of my mind or my subconscious, then those thoughts generate emotions. These emotions cause mounting distress and that distress then launches cravings. This sequence happens automatically and is unavoidable while my past and present issues circulate in my mind and this will *always* happen when my mind has spare processing capacity. So if I know this is going to happen then again, I can anticipate it, and prepare to minimise its impact. Idle time is to be avoided.

Anything that commands my full concentration will prevent my mind from having the spare capacity to work on unresolved issues, and this in turn will prevent unnecessary cravings. How to mitigate these issues is discussed later in this book but in the early days of recovery I needed to stop them from triggering me unnecessarily. So I prepared some things, ready to go, that would fully occupy my mind for these alone-times. The best of these were things that required a lot of hand-eye coordination. Simple entertainments weren't enough to keep the unwanted lines of thinking out of my mind so I had a range of tasks I could go to at a moment's notice. The most important thing was to know that alone-time was guaranteed to be troublesome and that as soon as I felt my mind wandering off on its own then I needed to fully occupy it, and quickly.

This section looked at why it was important to do three things early on: - occupy my mind during alone-time, fill my free time with activity that will lift my self-esteem, and radically change my routines to avoid the most triggering of locations. This last one meant opting out of some social activity for a while, but it was not forever. In time I would be able to go into places where alcohol was available and retain sufficient control that I did not drink, but that time was later. I needed the cravings to subside to a level that I was confident I could manage them before taking that risk. This meant I had to meet a lot of cravings and take the power from their triggers to lower the demand on my resolve before I could do that. But it was not forever. I had a plan and that plan slowly removed risk. I had to back off socially for a while but doing this was the very thing that would ultimately allow me to live freely in a world awash in alcohol. Early on I needed space between major cravings to prevent my resolve from becoming depleted. But almost every facet of my life had drinking triggers attached so there was no shortage of cravings that I *did* have to confront.

Overcoming cravings:

The previous chapter described how cravings work and it identified four characteristics of triggers that are important to know when it comes to stopping.

- Triggers lose strength (the craving they launch gets smaller) when I repeatedly do not drink in response to the cravings they launch.
- Cravings are automatically triggered by circumstances in which I have drunk before.
- Cravings are stronger when I am close to the triggering circumstance.
- Cravings have limited duration.

The first point in the list shows me the way out. The more I do this then the easier the road becomes. The second point shows me how to remove a lot of drinking triggers from my path so that I can lighten the load for a while and reduce the likelihood of my resolve being overwhelmed. The third and fourth points help me to get past the cravings that I *do* encounter.

There are many ways I can myself past carvings and five words in particular give me immediate direction: Describe, Distance, Delay, Distract and Deny.

Describe: I can immediately and dramatically lower the intensity of a craving by doing something incredibly simple. The very first thing to do when a craving comes on me is to acknowledge its presence. Next, if I can then identify the trigger that's been fired then I do so, and then I remind myself that the feeling is only temporary. I tell myself about these three things; out loud works best but in my head will do if that is all I can do in the circumstances. The conversation goes something like this: -

"Oh! There's a craving. It's probably just the time of day that set it off. It will do its thing and then move on".

This may sound like a trivial thing to do but it is not; it works. When I give my mind an explanation for what I am experiencing, and that it will end soon, then the craving becomes something that is to be expected rather than something alarming, and this lowers anxiety. There is nothing to be lost by talking to your brain like this so try it. It may feel a little odd at first but it takes very little effort to do and is a real "no loss" exercise; there is absolutely no penalty for trying it.

Urge surfing is an extension of this exercise. It is a technique used to observe and experience an urge without engaging with it. It is not about eliminating the urge; it is about allowing yourself to experience it calmly and not letting it build and dominate your thinking. The technique is to relax and let the urge go past rather than fight it and it works by deliberately calming the mind and then quietly observing the feeling without questioning or judgement of it. Anyone experienced in meditation or mindfulness will immediately know how to do this and there are plenty of self-help guides that will show you how. I couldn't always summon the calm to do this in the midst of a fierce craving, and I wasn't always in circumstances where I could stop what I was doing and be alone for a few minutes. But it worked at other times and it worked when I could effectively summon the calm required. Try it. If it helps then keep doing it, if it doesn't then nothing is lost. Whether or not urge surfing was possible or effective I still identified that I was having a craving and called it out. I could do this anywhere, anytime. It is an easy and effective way of lowering the impact of a craving but it took time to get into the discipline of doing it. Often I would be struggling with a craving before I remembered to do this, but I got better at it with practise. If I could get in early then this stopped the craving from climbing in intensity, and that is enough to do the job. Triggers lose their strength if they fail, but the cravings don't need to reach their peak to do this, they only have to be unsuccessful. So using this technique to prevent the craving from rising to a peak gets the benefit I want, to reduce the power of the trigger, but it reduces the distress involved in doing so.

Distance: Cravings are stronger when I am close to the circumstances of a trigger and there are many ways I can use this feature to help me. I can use it proactively to avoid some triggers, and I can use it reactively to lessen the intensity of some triggers that I *do* encounter.

It is extremely difficult to get sober if there is alcohol in the house and this feature of cravings explains why. If I know there is alcohol nearby then this will trigger almost continuous cravings and these cravings will be powerful because the source of that trigger is close. The great risk here is that confronting continuous and powerful cravings is exhausting and if it continues for too long then my resolve becomes depleted and resistance fails. This is why it is so important to remove alcohol from the house if that is possible. Buying alcohol also puts me close to it and I found it was just as impossible to manage. If the idea popped into my head that it might be good to have a bottle or two handy "just in case" then I needed to crush it immediately. If I buy alcohol then I am going to drink it; all that is undecided is when. So I stayed away from places that sold alcohol and wouldn't even pull into the car park of those places because once there the intensity of the motivation to go in and buy some would be even stronger. These actions used 'distance' to remove some triggers from my path for a while but I could also use this feature to lower the intensity and duration of other cravings.

The intensity of a craving is proportional to my closeness to its trigger, and this simple piece of knowledge is enormously instructive. I can reduce the intensity of a craving if I can identify its trigger and then move away from it.

Many people can avoid having alcohol at home but the world is awash with it and virtually every social occasion is accompanied by drinking. We can't avoid alcohol forever, indeed there are good reasons that we must not, but in the early days and weeks of stopping drinking it was extremely difficult for me to be in circumstances where people were drinking. Sometimes it was unavoidable, and while it wasn't impossible to negotiate these occasions, it *was* difficult and it *was* risky.

The first thing was to be aware that challenges were coming and not be blasé about this. Cravings are automatically triggered, so I have no way of stopping them, but forewarned is also forearmed. If I was going somewhere where there would be alcohol then I went there expecting to be challenged, and I went there knowing there was still something I had control over if I needed it: I could still control over how close I was to the circumstances of the trigger.

If I was at an event of some sort and the presence of alcohol was triggering me strongly then I could make those cravings lessen if I moved away. I could step away for a spell to make the cravings back off, or if necessary I could leave altogether. If I knew I was going to an event where there would be alcohol then I always made sure I had a way to leave if I needed to. Often the simple knowledge that I had a way to leave if necessary was sufficient to get me through a challenging occasion. Another thing I did to help myself on these occasions was to arrange to be accompanied by someone who knew that I wasn't drinking. Having someone there both provided encouragement to persevere and also made me very directly accountable in that time of heightened risk.

These actions will lessen or remove the craving but social events are about the occasion, not the alcohol, and this was a completely new concept to me. For years I regarded social gatherings as an opportunity to drink heavily and I needed to change my thinking because the other people weren't there for the drinking, they were there for the event. They weren't thinking about their next drink, they were enjoying the occasion. I was the only one fretting about alcohol and I was the one whose thoughts were preoccupied with drinking; the other people there could take it or leave it. The problem wasn't the event or the alcohol that was there. The problem was my reaction to it.

Distract and Delay: Cravings have limited duration. Knowing this I could grit my teeth and wait for the craving to end, but sitting and enduring a big craving is about the worst thing to do. If I sit there then the craving is going to direct my thoughts towards alcohol which will bring in other related thoughts, and pretty soon alcohol is all I can think about... and thinking about alcohol is enough to fire drinking triggers. Sitting and doing nothing while enduring a craving leaves my mind free to gather more and more drinking thoughts. This means that as soon as one craving fades then I will immediately trigger another. Sitting and trying to wait out a craving will make it more intense, last longer, and ensure that it is followed by another. There is a popular saying in recovery that "this too shall pass". But when it comes to cravings the best action isn't to wait for it to pass, a better action is to *do something* to make it pass.

If I choose the right sort of activity then I can occupy all the thinking capacity of my mind and leave no space for thoughts of drinking or other triggering ideas. If I can distract myself powerfully enough then the craving will pass while I am busy doing something else and I will not overcome one craving only to have it replaced by another.

The best activities for overcoming cravings were mentioned earlier; they are activities that require thinking and also hand-eye coordination. But to overcome a single craving I don't need this to be a big job or a long project, it only needs to last about 20 minutes. I don't need to get fancy about this, any task that requires these two things will do the job, so the possibilities are endless. Here are some of the things I used: - do some housework, tidy something, make something, cook something, go for a walk, jog, or swim, re-arrange something, clean something, go somewhere, write something, or call someone. I had a list of quick jobs I could do and I added to that list as fast as I crossed things off. The most difficult part of this was getting into the discipline of noticing the craving as early as possible, picking something from the list, *and then doing it.* Writing a list was easy when my head was in good shape but finding the motivation to do something when I really didn't want to do anything but feel sorry for myself was difficult. However, doing something off the list is what would make me feel better, and, odd as it seems, doing a chore is really good medicine for a craving. It completely changed the thought lines in my head and at the end of it I would get some satisfaction from knowing I'd done something worthwhile. Having a list of activities I could go to at short notice was important, but making myself start one of them was paramount.

The last thing on that list of distractions was unlike the others and that was to "call someone", and this was always a successful option. The reason this works is that talking to someone else makes me concentrate on what they are saying in order to respond, and this forces a change of subject on my brain. People had said "call me if you get into trouble" and when I was really struggling with a craving was the time they were talking about. They gave me their number for this very reason and if I rang then they knew why I was calling and were always willing to help. These conversations *always* carried me through a bad spell. It felt awful to make that call the first time I did it but it saved my bacon on several occasions. I built up a list of people that I could talk to easily when this happened and I used online communities to do the same thing.

Sometimes a craving would come on so fiercely that I couldn't concentrate on anything at all. I found that deliberate breathing helped with this. I would breathe in for four seconds and then breathe out for six. I'd concentrate on counting the breaths so I could hear the numbers really clearly in my head. I'd feel the air going in and then feel it go out. I'd hear the breath going in and then going out. If I kept this going for a few minutes, and kept concentrating on counting and on what I could hear and feel, then the panic would subside and I would regain enough composure to decide what to do next.

Cravings are inevitable. We can't avoid all triggers, nor do we want to because we need to meet cravings and overcome them to drive down their vigour. But there is plenty we can do to reduce the number we meet and to reduce their impact on us. But when all had failed and resolve had collapsed then there was still one more thing I was able to do with a little preparation.

Deny: If I lacked the means to acquire alcohol then even if I couldn't beat the cravings then I could still avoid acting on them, and I prepared for this possibility. There were things I could do that would prevent me from being able to drink *even if I wanted to*. Not having alcohol in the house (or in the garage, or under the house, or in the shed) was an obvious start on this but I had the good fortune to be living with a very supportive partner and this gave me some extra opportunities. She kept my keys and wallet so that I couldn't go anywhere without being accountable. I never carried cash, so anything I bought would show up on our bank statements. If I went out then I told her where I was going and for how long and that she could call me at any time. I kept my phone with me and turned on at all times, and if I needed to turn my phone off then I let her know why and for how long. Finally, and this was a big one, if we were going anywhere where there was going to be alcohol then she knew to intervene if it looked like I was going to take a drink and be firm with me about it. She also did something that I didn't discover until much later. Sometimes, if we were visiting friends for a BBQ or the like, she called them in advance and told them I wasn't drinking, and not to offer me alcohol. When we went to these places I wouldn't even be asked if I wanted wine or beer, I'd be offered something alcohol-free without any questions and this was a huge help.

Even if I had lived alone then there would still have been some ways to make myself accountable for the times that I was alone and able to buy alcohol. I could have asked people to confirm where I went and when I returned. I could pre-arrange to call people to do this or ask them to call me. If I was out, then I could have someone with me that knew they should stop me from drinking and give them permission to be assertive if necessary. I could assure them I would thank them for it later even if I protested at the time, because it is true; I would.

I had to assume that I *would* be confronted by a craving of such intensity that I wanted to drink, and I prepared in advance to deny myself the opportunity to do so if it happened. I also had to assume that I could not be trusted to stay away from alcohol in my time alone. I had failed to do so for years so I had no reason to expect that this had suddenly changed for the better.

This part of the book has looked at the main tools for coping with cravings and these are presented here as five D's; Describe, Distance, Delay, Distract and Deny. But there is one more way to get help with cravings that should not be overlooked.

Medication. The final word on things we can do to reduce the intensity of cravings goes to medication. There are all sorts of remedies touted as aids to stopping drinking and it is important to understand what will help, in what way they might help, and in what way they will not help. Dietary supplements will do nothing at all to alleviate cravings because cravings aren't caused by poor nutrition; they are caused by the way our brain responds to alcohol. But there are some remedies that may still provide some benefit for a while. Traditional remedies that lessen anxiety and improve sleep are both worth looking at but know that the relief given may be modest and that these two symptoms will right themselves as long as we stay away from alcohol. The symptoms they target are not cured by these treatments, because our body will fix these anyway given time, but they may give some temporary relief. For the most part the heavily promoted addiction "cures" are pharmaceutical nonsense, but there are some medications that are not. There are effective medicines available to address cravings and even if I didn't visit a doctor to talk about withdrawal then it would still have been worth doing so to explore these options.

There are three broad types of medication available to address cravings. The first is somewhat brutal as it will make us violently ill if we drink while taking it and Antabuse (Disulfiram) is the best known of these. What it does is it prevents the body from fully processing away alcohol and this causes a very severe hangover that lasts a long time. Having drunk on it once leaves a powerful motivation to not repeat the experience and this shows just how brutal the medicine is. One of the features of addiction is that we don't make alcohol-avoiding triggers very well, but the experience of drinking while on Antabuse is *so* unpleasant that it forces us to form one.

The next group of medications are those that reduce the intensity of cravings and Campral (Acamprosate) is the most well-known of these. Our brain changes the release rates of, and sensitivity to, several neurotransmitters to fend off the daily effects of alcohol. One of these changes is that glutamate activity is increased and Campral directly offsets that change. It eases the discomfort of early recovery by lowering anxiety and slowing the racing mind but there is limited evidence that it significantly changes our chances of staying sober in the long term.

The third group works directly on altering the way that the reward system operates. Naltrexone is the most well-known of these and it works by blocking the detection of dopamine in our brain. Drinking triggers release dopamine when they are fired but Naltrexone blocks that dopamine from being detected. The trigger is fired, dopamine is released, but the brain doesn't know that it is present and there is therefore no craving sensation. This removes the motivation to pick up a drink completely. A glass in front of us containing alcohol is no more interesting than a glass of water or milk. Taking naltrexone *and* *also* drinking progressively reduces the power of our drinking triggers because even though our brain is launching massive cravings they are undetected and there is no relieving "aaahhh", so the triggers think they have been unsuccessful and their vigour is lowered. This sounds like a wonder-drug but it has its drawbacks. It doesn't work for all people, and it can have some serious side effects that make it unsuitable for some.

There are medications we can take that will help when we stop drinking and it is foolishness to ignore any help that is available. But advice should be taken from a doctor, not an advert.

This chapter has looked at many ways we can help ourselves manage and negotiate cravings with a little knowledge. It has shown how we can methodically reduce the number of cravings we experience and how to reduce their intensity and duration. The aim is not to avoid all cravings because we must experience and overcome cravings in order for them to lose their vigour. The aim is to reduce and spread out the effect cravings have on us so that they don't overcome our resolve. At first I couldn't see the improvement but it was happening. I visualised this as a huge pile of rocks outside my door that I had to climb over to get in and out. Every time I went in or out I threw a few rocks off to the side. It took take time before any change became noticeable but the size of that barrier gradually got smaller. At first the scale of the problem appeared too big to change like this, but over time I could see some improvement and eventually I was able get in and out of the house with relative ease. This is what taking the power from triggers is like. It happens, it but it takes time.

Every time we meet and overcome a big craving is a battle won because the next craving to come from that trigger will be smaller and this means that we have just beaten the best it can throw at us. Celebrate these wins. Smile to yourself, do a little jig, have an extra piece of chocolate, whatever, but don't let the big achievements go unacknowledged. Every one of these is progress and every one is another step away from disaster and toward re-gaining control of our lives.

Keep going, because when people say; "Keep going! It gets easier" they are not just trying to encourage us; it is completely true.

Managing Resolve

Stopping drinking is a contest between my reward system demanding that I drink and my determination to stop, but it is not a fair fight. My reward system operates at a primal level that is invisible to me and it is armed with something I have no equivalent defence for and that is dopamine. This chemical is released in my brain with the express purpose of making me behave in certain ways, and in me it has become catastrophically linked to the acquisition of alcohol. Dopamine released by the reward system *motivates* me to drink, and that is its express purpose. This isn't me exercising poor choices; it is my brain explicitly enforcing a directive to drink.

Humans have executive cognitive functions that far exceed those of other animals. Animals have little capability when it comes to judgement, problem solving, or planning yet they live perfectly successful lives. This is because their actions are not random but are directed by their reward system. They don't plan their day by figuring out which direction they will go in search of food or what it is they'd like for lunch, they lack that capacity. It is their reward system that identifies a good feeding opportunity and directs them towards it. The reward system is what makes billions of creatures thrive and survive and it is the compelling power of dopamine that makes them do the things that will keep them alive. That same chemical urges me to seek out alcohol. It is enormously compelling and I have only my wits and force of will with which to try and overcome it. It is difficult to do once, it is very difficult many times in a row, and it is extremely difficult to do many times in a row for days on end.

Cravings are cyclical. They rise to a peak before fading away and resolve has a similar rising and falling pattern. If at any time I meet a craving at the top of its cycle when my resolve is at a low point then I risk drinking again. So it is essential that I not only reduce the intensity and frequency of cravings but also that I do whatever I can to keep my resolve high, because failure to do so invites relapse.

I notice the cravings because I feel them directly but I have no direct way of knowing the state of my resolve. This makes me inclined pay attention to the noisy part of the problem and ignore the silent part, but I do so at my peril. The acronym H.A.L.T is instructive in this respect. It is used to warn people of times at which they are at increased risk of relapse: Hungry, Angry, Lonely, and Tired. But only two of these (Angry and Lonely) are drinking triggers, the other two (Hungry and Tired) are times of low resolve. Relapse is just as likely to result from lowered resolve as it is from a heightened call to drink and this means that both sides of the equation are important. I am aware of the intensity of cravings but I have no awareness of the state of my resolve so it is easy to overlook this half of the problem. But I need to pay as much attention, if not more, to managing my resolve as I do to managing cravings. The more I can do to lift my resolve then the more secure I make my effort. Indeed, if my resolve is perpetually high then I will *never* be at risk of relapse. So this is the plan with resolve: - Do more of the things that will lift resolve and less of the things that deplete it.

The preceding chapter looked at ways to lower the intensity and frequency of cravings and this chapter looks at managing resistance to them. This is examined in three parts; things that destroy resolve and how do to reduce that, things that boost and replenish resolve and how to increase that, and how to maintain resolve over an extended period.

Contradicting the instructions from the reward system is a stern challenge and this challenge is not short-lived. At face value things should get easier as time passes but this is not quite what happens. Yes, it is true that the longer I go without a drink then the more cravings I overcome, and the more I make drinking triggers lose their strength then the more cravings will reduce in intensity. But I don't necessarily drink when I get an intense craving, *I drink when the intensity of the craving is greater than my will to overcome it.* The urge doesn't have to be powerful one, it only has to be greater than my will to resist it, and even a small craving can be sufficient to make me drink again if my resolve is low. Unfortunately there is something that changes resolve over time that it is spectacularly unhelpful in this regard, but the state of my resolve is invisible to me, so I don't notice it happening.

When I stop drinking then my drinking triggers slowly gave up their strength as I resist cravings but they never lose their power completely. If I stopped and checked myself I could see that this had happened because cravings that were once ferocious had become significant but were no longer debilitating. At the same time as this happened the defensive measures that my brain took to fend off alcohol were slowly removed and the feelings of anxiety, stress, fear, and hopelessness all began to recede. It seemed like I was winning the fight but there was another change that was very difficult to detect and this is that the urgency that drove my initial efforts to stop did not last; it faded away. It doesn't just sometimes fade, it is *guaranteed* to fade.

When I first stopped drinking I did so because I had reached a point that something *had* to change. This is often referred to as "the gift of desperation" whereby we reach such a low point that we become desperate to escape our trap and this gives us determination far beyond what we normally have. The gift of desperation gave me the extra boost that propelled me out of the jaws of the trap, but it could not last. As the time from my last drink increased then my brain removed more and more of the defensive measures it took against alcohol and my mood brightened dramatically. While it was wonderful to feel this release from despair it had an unwanted and invisible effect on my resolve because once I was relieved of hopelessness and depression then I ceased to be desperate, and when this happened then the extra strength that I got from that desperation disappeared too. As my distance from despair increased then my resolve to stop drinking plummeted, but I was completely unaware that this is what was happening.

Relapse in this period is perfectly common. In the early stages of becoming alcohol-free the effort is continuous and we have to be constantly vigilant and ready to fend off cravings as they come. Relapse at this later stage is often attributed to becoming "complacent" but that's not really what happens. What happens is that the problem changes and so does our perception of it. I no longer needed to live on continuous high-alert because the constant onslaught of devastating cravings had diminished and this coincided with a significant lift in my mood. The urgency of my cause faded and it was replaced by doubts about whether or not it was still necessary. It was, but the need to be alcohol-free was no longer blindingly obvious. I needed to be able to remain convinced that stopping drinking was still essential even though my life seemed to have improved dramatically.

It was vital that I maintained the belief that stopping drinking is necessary because without it my resolve would collapse, and this can't be stated any more plainly. If we neglect to maintain our resolve then we will drink again.

Things that destroy resolve.

I can sense my reward system in operation by noticing the urges it creates, but I have nothing to directly alert me to the state of my resolve. My resolve is low when whenever I am tired, hungry or run-down and I can do something about this if I notice it. But the simplest indicator of resolve is how I feel within myself. If I am emotionally low then my resolve is also diminished. At first there are so many things to stay on top of that I couldn't do them all, and I couldn't do them successfully all of the time, but there is one new skill that I *had* to acquire. I had to become continuously aware of my emotional state. It took time to build up this self-awareness but it is essentially the answer to the question "How am I?" If I was less than calm and relaxed then I needed to recognise that my resolve was low and I needed to do something about that because low resolve meant heightened risk. There were two things to do. I could do something to lift my mood if this was possible under the circumstances. But the more important step was to recognise that this was a time that I was vulnerable, and I that needed to lift my defences back up again. This shift into conscious awareness of risk immediately makes my mind alert to encroaching danger and ready to respond.

We only have our willpower and our wits to fight off acting on the cravings and picking up a drink. But when the cravings come fast and furious then this is exhausting. Fighting off cravings saps resolve and the previous chapter looked at many different ways we can reduce the impact of this. But cravings are immediately followed by something very destructive to resolve and that is self-sabotaging ideas. These are so damaging that the next chapter is devoted to this single subject. Becoming tired or emotionally low has already been mentioned as lowering resolve and ways to counter these are described on the following pages. But there is one thing that will destroy resolve more quickly and more completely than anything else, and that is picking up a drink.

I used to think that the advice "Don't pick up the first drink" meant that if I didn't have the first then I couldn't get drunk. But this is not the purpose of that advice at all. My problem isn't the fourth, fifth or even tenth drink, it is the first, because having one drink removes all objections to having another. The first drink collapses resolve. Once I have started drinking then my mind-set does an instant about-turn... "The damage is done now; I may as well carry on". If I take that first drink then my intent to have none is gone, and so too is any reason to hold back. So it was essential try everything in my power to avoid that first drink. Some things worked, some didn't, but there was one thing that worked every time, and that was to walk away. If things got too tough then I got up and walked out. It didn't matter if I was being rude; it was what needed to be done because if I stayed then I would drink again. Apologies could come later but what I needed to do in the moment was to leave. Nothing, absolutely nothing is more destructive to resolve than that first drink. So do whatever it takes to avoid it.

Things that boost or replenish resolve.

Just as there are many things that will reduce the demand on our resolve there are also many ways to replenish it and lift it up. Of all things I did there is one that stands head and shoulders above all others and that is becoming engaged in a recovery community. The research shows that the single most significant factor shared by people that achieve long-term sobriety is ongoing engagement in a recovery community. What matters statistically is not the particular type of group, but that contact with others in recovery is ongoing. I get numerous benefits from this but without them I am almost certain to fail. This may seem like an extreme statement, but it is very rare for anyone to become sober entirely on their own.

There are many different types of recovery group, both in-person and online, and while not everyone can take advantage of in-person meetings they are more powerful in terms of the gains we get. When I hear someone else's experience first-hand then it is far more compelling as it includes not only the words they say but also the full range of non-verbal cues. I get the nuances of their inflection and posture changes and I feel their emotion directly. This makes the insights I gain far more convincing. The strong recommendation here is that even if you don't think that group meetings are your thing, or if your circumstances make it difficult to get to them regularly, then go at least once. Everyone should go to at least one recovery meeting because there are some crucial things to observe there that can't be fully found remotely.

This book began by laying out the three fundamental beliefs we need to establish and uphold in order to stop drinking. These are that it is necessary, that it is possible, and that it is worthwhile. I can observe that it is necessary from my own experience of things getting worse and from my dwindling control. But I did not have similar insights into the other two; that it is possible, or that it is worthwhile. I can get these in a recovery meeting and if you only ever go to one meeting then you should do so for this reason. When I listened to people in recovery meetings then I heard the experiences of people at all stages of recovery and what became clear very quickly is that people that have stopped drinking for any significant period are calmer and they are happier. I could see direct evidence in these people that stopping drinking was not only worthwhile, but also that it was possible. I got something from the newer members too. From them I heard that a lot of their experiences were exactly the same as mine. I heard about anxiety, fear and hopelessness, and I heard about their racing mind, depression and restlessness. I suddenly discovered that I was not alone in this struggle and that these things were not unique to me; I saw that all alcoholics suffer from exactly the same problems. I saw that I wasn't the only person in the world struggling like this. I saw that alcoholism is very common and that so too is recovery. I saw that people had overcome it and this gave me something extraordinary... it gave me hope.

There should be no reason whatsoever I would not go to somewhere that could help me, but the prospect of walking into a recovery group was appalling. It felt like a very public confession of complete and utter failure. I half expected to find a room full of down and outs and derelicts and to be shamed for what I had become, but what I found was nothing even remotely like that. The people in the room were completely ordinary, like a random sample taken from a shopping mall. They had all been, or still were, in precisely the same predicament that I was in and none of them had any moral high-ground from which to judge me. I was not judged and I was not shamed. Instead I found find compassion, and I was encouraged not reprimanded. If there is a group nearby, even if it is some distance away, then you should steel yourself and go because you need to see what a recovered alcoholic looks like; it will help you immensely.

Pride was the barrier preventing me from getting help from people that understood this problem and had recovered from it. These people had achieved something that I could not do: they had stopped drinking. It was foolishness of me to deny myself access to such an invaluable resource and I should have done it years earlier but pride and my fear of being shamed prevented me from doing so. I had to deliberately redirect my thinking before walking into a recovery meeting to remind myself that when it came to overcoming alcoholism I was the novice and these people were the experts. They had done something that I could not and I needed to know what they knew. There was a lot said in those meetings and only some of it was relevant to me. Some was no doubt important to others in the room and some perhaps was important for me, but not at that time. I learned to let the parts that were not relevant to me slide past. I was not there to argue the merits or demerits of what was said, I was there to learn.

There are very many ways in which recovery meetings helped me and the main ones are listed here in no particular order: -

- Most of the talk was about what was going on inside our own heads and how to deal with that. I learned that the mental chatter, the stress, loneliness, fear etc. are not experiences unique to me; everybody else has (or had) them too. I was not going mad. These things are all a part of the alcoholic condition.
- I could get direct advice on how to deal with particular challenges: what would help and what would not. I did not have to waste time and effort on things that wouldn't work.
- Meetings changed the way I thought about addiction. It was nothing whatsoever to do with being a weak or a bad person.
- The convention was that before speaking everyone would begin with, "I am an alcoholic" and this had a very specific purpose. The aim is not to shame anyone, it is the opposite: it removes shame. What was therapeutic in this was the reaction from everyone else when I said it. The earth did not open up and swallow me and the audience did not recoil in horror, in fact, nothing happened at all. This is not what my brain was expecting the first time I said it because I was expecting to be shamed. But no judgement followed and my mind noted this. It learned that alcoholism is not shameful and this gave a huge lift to how I felt within myself.

- Meetings gave me affirmation that my course was the right one. Regularly seeing others that have recovered kept reassuring me that I was heading in the right direction and this repulsed the doubts that ran through my mind.

- An unexpected consequence of going to recovery meetings was that my self-esteem rose. Alcoholism is viewed as a weakness in general society and we are shamed for it. This is because our behaviour does not conform to that of the wider group. But in a recovery community our behaviour *is* the norm and therefore I did not feel like an outcast. This dramatically lifted how I perceived myself.

- In meetings I might be invited to talk about myself and my own experience. I got a lift from this that I didn't immediately identify but I felt its benefit nonetheless. It had nothing to do with what I said; it was to do with how the audience behaved. When I spoke in a meeting I was not interrupted. I spoke until I was finished. This is a sign of respect that is normally only given to people who are highly regarded and this did not go unnoticed by my brain. The fact that I was not interrupted until I was finished demonstrated to my mind that I was somebody significant, and again, this dramatically raised how I felt about myself.

- When I went to meetings regularly then the expectation was that I was not drinking in between them. This placed me under additional peer-pressure to stay alcohol-free and sometimes this added pressure was the very thing that stopped me from picking up a drink. This was an added resource that could prevent me from drinking but it also had a severe downside: if I drank again then I would not only feel that I had failed, but that I had failed in front of my peers. So the added impetus to stay alcohol-free would bite me if I *did* drink again. It helped, but this help came with risk.

- Meetings are sanctuary points and the value of this cannot be overstated. Stopping drinking isn't a brief challenge, it is ongoing, and most especially in the early days the effort can be exhausting. In-person meetings have a special quality about them and that is that while I was at them I could not drink: I was safe. If I was struggling then I could use this knowledge to help myself: all I had to do was to keep going until I got to the next meeting and then I would be safe again. This is something I had control over as I could choose how frequently I went to meetings. A key thing to recognise was that I could put these rest points into my journey as often as I needed them. My only challenge in this respect was to make sure that I took advantage of them and went, because when I least felt like going to a meeting was the time that I most needed to.

The single benefit I gained from meetings, that stands above all the others, is that all the items listed combined to give me something incredibly important: they restored my resolve. Some people in recovery groups become zealots for that particular recovery method but don't be put off by this because that is *their* truth. Statistically no recovery method is significantly better than any other. Some people get very enthusiastic about what worked for them and are dismissive of what didn't. But this doesn't mean that the other recovery methods didn't work, it means that they didn't work for them when they tried them. I certainly had this problem. For me no recovery effort succeeded until I needed it to. While I still had doubts about the necessity, possibility, or worth of stopping drinking then my attempt was certain to falter sooner or later regardless of the method I tried. But once I had fully accepted that I didn't know how to fix this myself then any recovery programme would probably have been successful.

For those that cannot or choose not to go to meetings it is still possible to get most of the benefits. There are many online ways to connect to a recovery community and that number of options is steadily increasing. These online groups allow me to benefit from the experience of others and I can use this to keep myself focussed and motivated. The groups that allow conversations with others in recovery and those that offer visual connection are the more useful because I get some empathy through these even if it is not as powerful as experiencing them in-person. The thing that cannot be completely gained remotely is the sanctuary effect of meetings but this can be found to some extent by engaging in an online recovery community and *staying* engaged. But regardless of the method I choose the research is clear that the single most significant thing I can do to avoid relapse is to stay actively involved in some sort of recovery community. It keeps me reminded of what I am trying to achieve and it maintains my resolve. But recovery groups aren't the only way to lift resolve; there are many other ways that I can directly manipulate it.

- When I am struggling then talking to another alcoholic always helps enormously because they understand me. It is a quick and easy way to get stood back up again.
- I can deliberately put joy in my life. I can put a highlight in my life every day. It doesn't have to be

anything fancy, just something to look forward to and something that is just about me.

- I can have sweet things and snacks handy to give myself small treats as I go through my days.
- Getting outdoors always helps. Being in nature recharges me, and especially elevated places, places with a distant horizon, and views across water. Any is of these is good, all is better.
- I can make myself accountable by telling someone I am doing this. This raises the penalty on me if I drink but it puts one more obstacle between me and alcohol.
- I can do something to help someone else. This seems an odd thing to put in a list of things that help resolve but it works. We evolved to live in communities and one of the things our brain does is it rewards us when we do something that benefits the group even though there is no direct benefit to ourselves. My brain gives me an inner feel-good sensation of satisfaction when I help others and feeling good about myself strengthens resolve.
- Positive thinking. This is a simple exercise I can do that will always make me feel good. It works best when I am in a moving scene, like being out for a walk, or in traffic, or on a bus or train. I look around and think something good about every person,

object or activity that my eyes come to rest on. After 15 minutes or so of this I am fizzing with positivity and enthusiasm and my resolve is restored.

There are many ways in which I can manage my resolve, both to reduce it becoming depleted and to top it back up again, but the challenge is not short. When I first set out I was powered by the extra determination I got from desperation but this did not last forever; it receded as my life ceased to be so distressing. But the challenge did not stop at the same time, it kept going. It dropped in intensity but it continued for months, even years, and in truth I am never completely free of it. I might remove all the symptoms of alcoholism and no longer notice their impact on a daily basis, but if I stop doing the things that keep me well then they will return.

Maintaining resolve over an extended period.

I didn't suddenly "get it" and then forever after remain committed to not drinking. After I managed to stop drinking for a month or so then all the defensive measures of alcohol-tolerance that my brain put in place slowly reversed out. The racing mind, fear, stress, and anxiety all faded away and the urgency of my cause faded with them. Once I was feeling well again then the initial desperation that propelled my effort disappeared. I still got cravings, strong and frequent, but they weren't debilitating like they once were. They still took deliberate effort to overcome and I was aware of their constant presence but otherwise things were OK. This is when the self-sabotaging lies really kicked in.

I have to keep the three pillars of my recovery firm: that stopping drinking is necessary, possible and worthwhile, and they are constantly being challenged. If I don't work to keep my commitment firm then the self-sabotage will eventually get the better of me and I will drink. This is consistent through all stages of recovery, but there is a perversity about this. The longer I go and the more successful I am in taking power from my cravings then the less necessary this effort appears to become. This makes the sabotaging lies become more plausible and I have to maintain my resolve to combat this.

I never reach the point that I have beaten alcohol; I am susceptible to addiction and I remain vulnerable for my whole life. I can remove all of its symptoms but I am never cured. What I *do* achieve is I bring my addiction into remission, but if I completely stop treating the condition then it will return. What makes this so difficult is that I lack a direct way to know how secure my resolve is at any particular moment and I have to develop a new skill to determine this. The important thing to be aware of is that my vulnerability is permanent and that I become more at risk of drinking again whenever my emotions begin to slide. This is when the self-sabotage is most effective. It is when "a drink will make you feel better" sounds convincing, and it is when I am far enough from my last drink that the penalties of drinking are long driven from my memory. I needed ways to remember why it was so important that I stopped in the first place, and I needed to help myself continue to do what was needed to stay free from alcohol. I had to keep doing what was working even when there no longer seemed any need to do so. So what could I do to help myself with this?

When I made paying attention to recovery a routine activity rather than something I did when the situation demanded it then I built myself a recovery tool that was enduring. By establishing a routine early on, when the need was obvious, then I gave myself something I could continue easily and it gave me a known position to move back to if things became difficult again. Precisely what a daily routine should look like is entirely individual and it is individual for a very good reason. There is no "one way" that will work for everyone because we are all motivated differently. Some find checklists and schedules helpful, some write journals, some meditate, and some find strength in their faith. All of these will help someone maintain a consistent course but not all will work for everyone. What I needed to do was to establish a daily routine that suited my own motivators but also one that was not so demanding that I couldn't keep it going for a long time. Regardless of what I do or when I do it the crucial component of my routine is to ensure that I think about my recovery every single day.

I am going to describe my routine here. This is not a suggestion of how it should be done; it is only here as an example. We each need work out what will work for ourselves and what we can sustain over a long timescale, but here's a tip: keep it *really* simple because it is something that you need to be able to keep going *every day*.

My morning routine is to use my shower time to set myself up for the day. It always starts the same way with the mental statement "I am an alcoholic". This isn't a damaging thought to me at all because I attach no shame to it. What I find helpful about it is that it reminds me that I have to do something about this problem and it sets off a train of thoughts: - I have a condition called alcoholism. It can't be cured but it can be put into remission and kept there. What do I need to do about this today? What are the challenges I can expect today? I don't try and control the direction of the thoughts that come and every day they will run differently depending on how I am feeling and what the day is likely to hold. The key thing is that I start my day thinking about recovery. When I began I stayed connected to recovery by going to meetings regularly. When I first set out I knew that I could not trust myself and I needed to keep my sanctuary points close so initially I went to recovery meetings every day. Over time the frequency I needed meetings reduced but that need never goes away completely and even after some years of continuous sobriety I still need frequent contact with others in recovery to maintain my resolve. To do this I make sure I engage with at least one other alcoholic every day. This is a firm rule I have with myself. If I do not do this then I have learned that I will begin to slide emotionally. I do it every day without exception.

This is the extent of my routine. It is not so demanding that I can't maintain it and it does what I most need: it reminds me every day that I still have a problem that requires me to *do* something. It may not be much that I have to do, but equally it is never quite nothing. This routine works for me but people are unique and differently motivated. It is important to organise your own routine around what motivates you and also what you will be able to maintain over long period. If you meditate then use that, you will gain great advantage from being able to observe how the threads of addiction flow in your mind. If you write then journal about recovery because journaling allows you to directly record progress and turning back the pages will remind you how important it is to keep going. If you are a person of faith then include recovery in your routine of devotions: ask for help, guidance, and give thanks. If you have an exercise routine then use that as a time to think about recovery. However we organise our routine is unimportant, what matters is that we find a way to think about recovery every day because that is what keeps motivation up and that is what allows us to keep our course true in the long term. And if things start going off the rails then the routine is a point of safety to return to, because we know that while we followed it then things went well.

If recovery meetings are not a part of your routine then you are missing out on several things that will help you, but you can provide at least one of these for yourself. One of the many benefits of meetings is that I saw people that were new in recovery. These were people who were desperate and they kept me reminded of just how bad things really were; how raw and distressing life had been. It really *was* bad, but distance from despair hides that from me. If I am not having this memory refreshed at meetings then I need to find other ways to do this and I do this through online engagement. It works. It keeps me reminded of why I had to do this in the first place and that I need to keep doing the things that keep me well.

The time I least feel like working on my recovery is the time that I most need to and this is an unfair twist in the path but it is what happens. If I do really well then I will be on top of managing cravings and resolve and I will feel fine. But feeling well makes the effort I am putting in seem redundant. I don't notice a problem when it is absent, but if I don't do the things that *keep* it absent then it will return. It is unfair but success breeds the conditions for failure, and keeping on doing what's working, even though it seems unnecessary to do so, is one of the many disciplines to master. The other reason I stop wanting to work on my recovery is much harder to overcome and it is that I just don't feel like it. I get like this when I'm feeling low and out of sorts with the world and I really just can't be bothered. This puts up massive red flags for me. When I'm feeling down and tired is when I least want to do the things that will help me, but it is also when I most need to do them. It takes huge effort to pull out of this and of all the disciplines in recovery to this was one of the hardest to master, but failing to do so sets me on a path to drinking again.

All of recovery is built on improvement. We progress, we slip back a little, we learn what does and doesn't help, and our recovery becomes slowly more robust. The aim is progress not perfection. The bottom line is that if we keep working at it then we keep improving our chances of success. It works if we work at it; but it doesn't if we don't. Keep going.

Self-sabotage

The reward system sits in the subconscious part of my brain and it operates entirely automatically and invisibly. There is no conscious thought involved in its operation and it is not even directly connected to the parts of my brain that deal with decision-making and judgement. So while my higher mental functions may have reached the conclusion that I should stop drinking my reward system didn't get the memo: it still wants me to drink. My conscious decision to stop has no impact whatsoever on the reward system. It still directs me to drink every time I encounter the circumstances of a trigger and this process happens invisibly and automatically; I have no means of turning it off. But cravings, regardless of their intensity, do not come on their own; cravings are always accompanied by ideas that encourage me to drink. My conscious mind *always* presents a supportive justification of the craving. It does this because the dopamine enforced instruction has come from the reward system and instructions from the reward system are important and to be acted on because they are to do with survival. So whenever I get a craving to drink then I also get an accompanying rationalisation of why I should do what it urges. In this respect my condition is every bit as cunning, creative and deceitful as I can be, because *I* am a component of the condition. Self-sabotage isn't imaginary. It is perfectly real and it is in every way my intellectual equal. This is why it is so convincing and this is why it is so dangerous. I must counteract it because left unchallenged it will steadily corrode all resolve.

Self-sabotaging thoughts are another reason that normal drinkers can't understand alcoholics because they have a completely different experience. They get mental messages in support of cravings too, but they don't just get prompts from drinking triggers, they get them from alcohol-avoiding triggers too. If it is an inappropriate time for them to drink then they are motivated away from alcohol and get a thought like "I've got to drive later". They are actively persuaded away from alcohol, but I never am. I am always, and only, encouraged to drink, and to drink now. I don't have alcohol-avoiding triggers so the accompanying thoughts I get always present drinking as a good idea and never a bad one. But what makes this even more serious is that these ideas aren't only generated when I get a *severe* craving, they come when I get *any* craving. This means that the reducing intensity of cravings over time does not stop the sabotaging thoughts from coming. My conscious mind responds to the instruction coming from my reward system regardless of how loudly it is shouted. Thoughts of drinking are prompted by cravings, large or small, and while I was still drinking then I got these virtually non-stop. This is how my mind became preoccupied with drinking, from my waking thoughts to my last, and this does suddenly stop when we stop drinking.

The great challenge for me was that these alcohol-encouraging ideas did not go away once I'd decided to stop drinking. The reward system still urged me to drink every time a trigger was fired and each time that happened then a thought would pop into my mind to explain why drinking now was a good idea. When I first set out to stop drinking it was the intense cravings that were my biggest challenge. But as the cravings lessened in intensity then the mental chatter encouraging me to drink again became my main risk and I learned that I must not ignore it. If I do not challenge these ideas as they come then they erode the foundations of my recovery because most of the self-sabotage is directed at the foundations of recovery; that stopping drinking is necessary, possible and worthwhile.

Sabotaging thoughts are not only frequent they are also plausible. This happens because they are lies built upon other lies, and the main culprit here is my memory. I have two deep settings which determine which way triggers get formed in me: - I value the prize more than the risk that comes with it, and I value something now much more highly than I value something later. But these thresholds don't just determine whether I make alcohol-avoiding triggers or not, they are also used to determine what information is to be kept as a memory and what is to be discarded.

I remember the good things about drinking far more strongly than I remember the bad things, and my memory doesn't care much about what happened later so it only links it very weakly to drinking. My memory records the good times and laughter, but not the disastrous consequences. It strongly remembers that "drinking is fun" but it glosses over the anxiety, stress, hopelessness, shame, guilt and it doesn't connect the later consequences to my drinking the night before. Above all things my memory tells me that "drinking is fun!" This may have been true once but it wasn't in the end: drinking was lonely, and miserable. When my head flooded with reasons why I should drink then my memory was the bogeyman that silently confirmed "it's true, it's true; do it!" This biased memory is why I don't learn from my mistakes when it comes to drinking, because the mistakes aren't well linked to alcohol in my memory. But there is one more feature of memory that works against me.

There is a psychological phenomenon called "Fading Affect Bias" and this gradually distorts my perception of the past: memories that are associated with negative emotions are faded more quickly than those associated with positive emotions. This makes looking back on something that happened a while ago seem better than it actually was, because all the downsides are diminished. The joke "nostalgia isn't what it used to be" reflects this very phenomenon but when it came to memories of my drinking it wasn't funny. My recall of bad outcomes from drinking was already poor, but FAB faded it almost out of sight.

Distance from despair and FAB are not the same thing. Distance from despair describes how my mood gradually lifts over time as the effects of alcohol-tolerance reverse out. This leaves me happier but takes away the boosted determination I gained from the 'gift of desperation'. FAB is different in that it distorts my perception of the past making it appear more fun than it actually was. It takes away what meagre memories I have of the misery and downsides of drinking and this enhances the good parts. When I stop drinking then my memory tells me that I am missing out on fun. But my memory omits to tell me how bad things were and it does not remind me that my life was so miserable that I was desperate for escape. When it comes to alcohol my memory is falsely optimistic, and incredibly so. If I am asked to imagine myself drinking in a drinking scene then I always get a positive memory first and never a bad one. My primary recall of drinking is always of good times and fun and it is never of all the awful things I said, caused, or that happened to me. It seems that "drinking is fun!" is engraved in my mind in the largest possible font, but it isn't true. If drinking was really as good as my memory tells me then how come I became so desperate to stop? It is lies upon lies upon lies, and these lies have to be challenged or they take hold.

My memory isn't faithful when it comes to alcohol, and this "always good" representation of drinking verifies the self-sabotage. When an idea comes into my mind in support of a craving then it is compared to what I know in my memory and a conversation starts up with all manner of supporting information cascading in. So what starts as an urge supported by an idea ends up being a craving accompanied by a barrage of chatter telling me why drinking now is such a good idea. It is all lies and the lies sound really convincing because they are confirmed by my own memory. But I can actively do things to alter those memories. I can't erase old ones and create new ones, but I *can* alter the likelihood that a bad memory of alcohol will be recalled instead of a good one.

Memories are stored information and our brain makes commonly referenced information faster to access. Just like triggers become more powerful through repeated success a remembered detail becomes more accessible the more often it is recalled. Memory is made faster by repetition. In my memory "drinking is fun" has been reinforced so many times that I know it more confidently than any other fact. False facts cannot be removed, what has become known cannot become unknown, but they *can* be superseded by newer information. We do this all the time with other facts and we can exactly the same thing to our drinking memories. We don't forget old pieces of information that have been demonstrated to be incorrect, they are still there, but our mind reduces their importance and if new information is sufficiently well reinforced then we get that first instead. This simple piece of knowledge shows me how I can help myself change the way my memory works in relation to self-sabotaging ideas. I can change my memory from always presenting drinking as "fun". I can reduce its bias.

So far this book has laid out a simple plan to deal with cravings and another for manging resolve, and now comes the plan for dealing with a biased memory. I can't remove the memory that says "drinking is fun", but I *can* reinforce the memories that demonstrate "no it wasn't!" It is a very simple technique, but like so many other things in addiction simple is not the same as easy. I selected three incidents from my past that were direct consequences of drinking and that were also absolutely heinous. These were the three most awful things that had happened as a consequence of my drinking and they were the three memories that most made me squirm inside when I recalled them. I then set about deliberately strengthening these. I gave each of these memories a single keyword to remember it by and then remembered that three keyword phrase. Then, and this is the hard part, whenever I had some rose-tinted vision of wanting a drink I chanted the three keywords in my head and spent a moment dwelling on each of them recalling its event. This slowly strengthened the counter-point in my memory to "drinking is fun!" It was a slow discipline to master and I often missed a chance to exercise those memories, but every time I succeeded then my memory's encouragement of drinking slowly grew weaker. It isn't an easy discipline to engage, but it works, and by steadily strengthening bad memories of drinking it becomes less frequent that having a drink seems such a convincing idea.

My subconscious mind actively works against my efforts to stop drinking and I have to recognise this as a fact of life. I can't believe everything I think. When I experience a craving then my mind automatically serves up ideas that support drinking and the sole purpose of these ideas is to make me drink again. It is a mechanism that I can't prevent from operating and I have only limited means to alter what it throws into my consciousness. But the sabotaging ideas don't just come and then pass; their effect is cumulative. Self-sabotaging ideas work in exactly the same way as propaganda. Even though the information is false, if I hear it enough times then I start to believe that it is true. This means that if I let these ideas run freely then they will become increasingly more convincing until resolve is overcome and I will drink. It is essential to find ways to counteract their effect because if I don't then they are a highway to relapse.

Cravings all have one thing in common and that is that they are created in error because my reward system makes a terrible mistake when it comes to alcohol. Alcohol is *not* beneficial to me, it hurts me, and the cravings I get do not aid my survival, they are harmful to it. All cravings are created in error, and therefore all ideas supporting cravings are also false, and this is a key piece of information: all self-sabotaging ideas are false. They are lies, and lies, when they are proven to be false, lose their conviction.

What I have in my favour with self-sabotaging lies is that there are not too many ways to make my drinking appear rational. My drinking was utterly destructive in the end so the positives are few and far between and the range of plausible lies that can be dreamed up to make it appear good are quite limited. The number of the deceptions is quite small and most alcoholics experience the same ones. Here are some of the most common lies. They don't always present themselves in exactly these words but many of these themes will already be familiar.

– "Just one won't hurt"
– "No-one will know"
– "You've done well, you deserve a drink"
– "Forever!"
– "Perhaps I wasn't that bad"
– "I can probably control it now"
– "A drink will make me feel better"

These, and similarly damaging ideas are definitely coming and the plan for these is to crush them as they arrive. The task is not to negotiate with them, the task is to confront them and dismiss them as incorrect because this is what will stop my brain from continuing to present them. Every plausible seeming reason that I should drink is untrue so the challenge is to identify the lies and expose them as false. But not only do I know that self-sabotaging thoughts are going to come; I also know what most of them look like. So I can anticipate and prepare for their arrival. If I know in advance the way in which each idea is false then I can take the conviction from each one as it arrives.

"Just one won't hurt" This justification is a lie because one *will* hurt. If I have one drink then I have placed myself in the presence of alcohol and this will cause drinking triggers to fire constantly. Not only does the next craving (and accompanying sabotaging thought) come as soon as my glass is empty it comes with incredible intensity because the power of the craving depends on how close I am to the trigger, and I have put myself somewhere where I am surrounded by them. But not only does the challenge of cravings rise, the strength of my resolve simultaneously collapses. This has already been described: having one drink removes all objections to having another.

But "just one" is also a ridiculous suggestion; when did that ever happen? I never drank "just one" so why on earth would it be any different now? I spent years proving to myself that I have no control over my drinking once I start, so one drink will lead to another.

There is no such thing as "just one" and there never was. I can't do that. If I could do "just one" then I wouldn't have this problem in the first place. Having one drink removes all objections to having another and that is the trap. The lie is "one"... because it won't be. It never was, and it never will be.

"No-one will know" This justification is a complete misdirect. The "no-one will know" justification is not about alcohol it is about shame, or rather the avoidance of it. The problem was that alcohol was destroying my life, whereas shame is about being *seen* to be drinking in ways that others don't approve of. The idea is that if I drink and don't get seen then I can avoid being shamed and this is the motive that drives me to drink secretly. But that is not the problem! My problem is that drinking is destroying me, not whether or not it is seen. "No-one will know" means that I can avoid some shame but it does not make drinking OK because drinking is disastrous for me whether it is seen or not. This is not a reason why I should drink. It is at best a feeble excuse; but mostly it is irrelevant. The response to "no-one will know" is "So what? The damage will still get done"

"You've done well, you deserve a drink" This idea suggests that drinking is some sort of reward for good behaviour. But having a drink is *not* a good way to reward myself for not drinking, it is a stupid one. Anxiety, fear, shame, guilt and remorse are not rewards but these are precisely what I get if I drink again. But my memory doesn't tell me this and I have to actively remind myself of it. A drink is not good for me; it is bad for me. Alcohol is not a reward, it is a punishment, and that is the lie.

"Forever!" This strikes directly at the idea that stopping drinking is possible. My experience of stopping drinking was that it was impossible; I could do it for a short while, but not in the long term, so "forever" seems to be an utterly unobtainable goal. It was absolutely inconceivable that I would *never* drink again; not even once, forever. This idea leads me to expect that failure is inevitable, in which case why delay? If I am going to drink at some point in the future, then why am I torturing myself now? I may as well go and have a drink and put an end to the struggle.

This is an appealing idea, but it is entirely false. There are two ways to counter this idea and the first is to be found in people that have been in the same position and recovered, and there are *a lot* of these people. Read books, listen to podcasts, listen to other peoples' direct evidence in recovery groups; all of these sources confirm that stopping drinking is perfectly possible. But there is another more complete way to dismiss this lie and that is that "forever" is not what I am trying to achieve. I am not trying to give up forever... I can't possibly know the future with that degree of certainty. What I am doing is I am not drinking *today*. Tomorrow is a different problem, and the day after, and Christmas, and birthdays, and New Year and so on. I can deal with those as I get to them but they are not the challenge yet. The challenge is not forever, the challenge is now! All I have to do is not drink for the rest of the day and that is something that I know I *can* do. I know I can do this because I've done it before, therefore it is not impossible.

A catch-cry of all recovery methods is "One day at a time" and it is so for good reason. "One day at a time" tells me to keep my horizon close. So I need to keep my head out of the future and deal with what is in front of me right now; the future isn't here yet. I can't guarantee that I will not drink "forever" and that is the doubt that this lie relies on, but I do know that "today" is achievable. Dismiss forever. Forever is not the challenge. The challenge is to not drink today.

"I can probably control it now." No I can't. I never could control my drinking and I never will because I lack the means to do so. At the deepest level my problem isn't that I lost control of how much I drank, it was that I never had the means to control it in the first place. Stopping drinking for a spell may make the severity of the cravings lessen and I might feel happier within myself but that doesn't mean I have gained any control. It is that the challenge has become less demanding and the urgency less apparent. Stopping for a while doesn't remove the drinking triggers and replace them with alcohol-avoiding triggers. All the drinking triggers are still there and my mind still lacks the means to make effective alcohol-avoiding triggers. I haven't regained the ability to control my drinking and I never will. I have already proved that I can't control my drinking countless times and if I drink then I will only end up proving it once again. I can't control my drinking and that is why I had to stop. Control has not changed; it is the challenge that has become less severe. I can't control my drinking because I lack the means to do so and I always will because it is written into my DNA. To suggest otherwise isn't just a lie, it is a very dumb one.

"Perhaps I wasn't that bad" Who I am trying to kid? This lie stands or falls on my biased memory. When I visualise drinking then I get images of good times and laughter. But that isn't the reality of what happened. What is not offered to me is all the awful stuff; the terrible things I did, the bad things that happened because of my drinking, the fact that I kept repeating the same mistakes, and so on. I don't get shown how all the things I did filled me with guilt, shame and remorse, and I don't get how hopeless and trapped I felt. All of this is in my memory but it isn't presented to me as strongly as the good bits, which in truth had become few and far between. Yes, I *was* that bad. All I have to do to prove this is to think of the top 10 worst things that happened because of my drinking and remind myself of how these made me feel because that was the strongest motivator to stop. My memory is reluctant to give up these details, but they are there. As soon as I bring back to mind the brutal truth about my drinking then I prove to myself very quickly that I really *was* that bad, and that is why I had to stop. It really was that bad, and to say otherwise is a complete nonsense.

"A drink will make me feel better." This last justification is also the most insidious and it gets attached to *all* of my emotional drinking triggers. This one is the most challenging to deal with because it is true: a drink *will* make us feel better. It is still built on a lie, but exposing the lie doesn't help me as much as might be expected. The lie in this statement is hidden in the timing. Yes, a drink will make me feel better *now*, but I will feel far worse *later*. But this is the weak point in my armour because I intrinsically don't care much about later; a drink now is important to my brain but the later penalty isn't. To expose this lie I have to *make* myself think about later. What I do is to deliberately force my mind to fully recognise the later consequences of drinking and the trick here is to "play it forward". When the idea comes up "a drink will make you feel better" then I play the scene forward in my mind to find out what happens next. One drink leads to two drinks leads to a bottle and then everything goes to hell on a handcart from there. What happens next? And what happens after that? Playing it forward uses my own experience to show me that yes, a drink might seem like a good idea right now, but it is going to end in disaster. It is a way of forcing me to properly recognise the down-sides of having a drink that I won't fully recognise naturally.

Self-sabotaging thoughts are inevitable and if I don't push back against them then they will eventually convince me to drink again. But like so many things in addiction, knowing what to do is far easier than actually doing it. Nothing in recovery is passive. I have to step in and correct it when my mind is doing the wrong thing, but I can only do this when I notice that something has gone awry in the first place. I have to detect the wayward thought and then actively dismiss it as false. Sometimes I go a long way down a rabbit-hole before I recognise I am in one, but when I do I can expose the lie and reject it forcefully. When I consistently denounce the lies then my mind recognises that they are failing and after a while it stops bothering to present them.

We can't prevent the self-sabotage thoughts from coming because they are a direct response to cravings, but we *can* steal their conviction, so that is the plan. Recognise the lies and denounce them as they come. They exist *only* to make us drink again, but they only work if we believe them and they have no power over us if we don't.

Don't believe everything you think about alcohol because half of it isn't true. Expose the lies and steal their persuasiveness.

Emotional Triggers

If we drink frequently and heavily then our brain's performance becomes routinely impaired, and it changes the way it operates to try and offset this. The principal action of alcohol on the brain is that it slows it down. This is what causes me to talk nonsense, lose balance, get sleepy, slur my words, and so on. My brain tries to counteract this by speeding up both my brain and body. It accelerates how fast I am thinking, it tries to wake me up, and it gets my blood circulating faster to try to get me moving properly. Some of this is done with neurotransmitters (chemicals passed between nerve cells in our brain) and some with hormones (chemicals in the bloodstream that tell our organs what to do). These chemicals are released to combat the slowing effects of alcohol and I can feel their lingering effect when I start to sober up: - I have a pounding heart, and my over-excited nervous system makes me tremble. But if I drink frequently then these chemicals aren't only released in response to alcohol they are also released the whole time in anticipation of it, and my brain and body become persistently over-stimulated. I remain over-stimulated until I drink again. Once I drink frequently and heavily then my brain and body are over excited and I need alcohol to return them to their "normal" state. This is the real effect of becoming alcohol-tolerant. It doesn't simply mean that I can drink more without it showing, it means that my body has adapted to tolerate more alcohol before becoming functionally impaired. But some of these changes it makes to do this have a terrible effect on us emotionally.

Alcohol slows the brain down but the other major effect of alcohol is that it makes me artificially happy, carefree, and socially confident. Drinking causes endorphins and serotonin and to be released and these are what cause the mood change. But when I drink frequently then my brain recognises that it is getting more fun and sociability than it ordered and it slows down release of these chemicals to try to correct this. This in turn causes me to be less sociable, less carefree, and less happy at the times when I am *not* drinking.

When I drink frequently then the changes in the way that my brain works make me feel normal while I am drinking but I feel anxious, restless, irritable, unhappy, and socially shy when I am not. My accelerated mind churns, tumbles, and races over all of my problems and anxiety climbs. All of these symptoms are soothed by alcohol, because alcohol slows my mind down, calms me, and cheers me up... so I drink. But once I take a drink to escape these emotions then my brain recognises this improvement and it creates a drinking trigger for each of them.

Once my brain has adjusted how it works to defend itself against the effects of alcohol then I become anxious, agitated, irritable, and miserable whenever there is no alcohol in my system. But each of these emotions is a drinking trigger so I end up being triggered to drink whenever I am sober! I am motivated to drink to relieve these symptoms but drinking more makes my brain adapt these defensive measures even more strongly. When this happens I become locked into a self-reinforcing cycle whereby drinking eases the emotions that are *caused* by drinking, but drinking more only intensifies these emotions further.

This is the second self-reinforcing loop of addiction. The first one is that in the absence of alcohol-avoiding triggers our drinking triggers increase in strength without limit. The second loop is that frequent drinking lowers our mood, which we drink to relieve, which then lowers our mood even further, which makes us drink even more. The first sets my course and the second locks that course into place.

Just as it took time for my drinking triggers to gain in strength it also took time for my emotional decline to develop and I didn't readily make the connection between the two, in fact I got it back to front. The longer I drank frequently then the more anxious, stressed and depressed I became. My life seemed hard and I drink for relief from that. A common thought was "if you knew how I felt then you'd drink too!" We might once have drunk to relieve some persistent hardship or to escape the distress of some traumatic event, but once we engage that second feedback loop of addiction then we become triggered to do so whenever we are sober. This causes our drinking to escalate further and the anxiety, fear and hopelessness intensify. If we carry on drinking then we become so depressed that we can no longer even drink enough to make ourselves happy and alcoholics often describe this as "alcohol stopped working for me". The distress in our lives builds and many go to doctors seeking relief from depression, but what we actually need is relief from alcohol. When I was still drinking I didn't realise that the two were so completely linked.

Understanding how addiction forms and what drives it means that I can focus my effort where it will bear fruit instead of chasing false causes. I did not become an alcoholic simply because alcohol is an addictive substance; that is not the reason at all. Yes, alcohol is addictive, but it is not addictive to everyone. If a normal drinker is using alcohol for relief from some adverse circumstances then their alcohol-avoiding triggers will steer their drinking back to a moderated state if that distress ceases. They have an "off" switch, but I do not and I never will. I didn't choose for it to be this way and I didn't make it this way, it just is. My problem isn't caused by other people, places or things. It is not caused by what happened in my past, it is not alcohol advertising that makes me addicted, nor is it simply that alcohol is addictive. Other people have problems, other people see the same media promotion of alcohol as I do, and other people drink the same stuff as I did, but they do not all become addicted. I did because I don't make alcohol-avoiding triggers, and all of the other problems of addiction compounded out from there.

When I realise that the problem is within my own mind then I see too that the solution also lies with me. Changing other people does not fix the problem, changing jobs does not fix the problem, moving somewhere else does not fix the problem, and winning the lottery will not fix the problem. All these things do is move me away from a few triggers for a while but wherever I go and whatever I do I will quickly create new triggers for my new circumstances and soon I will be back exactly where I was. The only way to escape alcoholism is to remove the vigour from my drinking triggers and the way to achieve this is by making them consistently fail to deliver alcohol. If I am are able to sustain my effort to stop drinking then all of the defensive changes that came with alcohol-tolerance become unnecessary and my brain will steadily remove them. The first of these noticeable changes is that sleep returns and after that then anxiety fades and then the agitated churning of my mind calms down. There is nothing I have to do to make the fear, anxiety, restlessness, racing mind and hopelessness disappear. My brain will correct all of these itself... all I have to do is not drink!

Once they are formed then drinking triggers remain in place for life; they are never forgotten. I can reduce their power to a point that the cravings they launch no longer interfere with my day, but unfortunately this general behaviour of triggers is not the whole story when it comes to emotions. Regular triggers are fired by a specific location or occurrence that relates to alcohol, but my emotional triggers are fired depending on how I feel *regardless* of what has caused the emotion. Anything that lowers my mood or brings on an adverse emotion will fire a trigger that launches a craving. The normal remedy of moving away from the location of the trigger will not work because the trigger moves with me: *I* am the trigger. And while a regular drinking trigger will launch a craving that rises to a peak and then passes my emotional triggers may not. For example, if I have a trigger associated with feeling down, a "poor me" trigger so to speak, then it will launch an urge to drink whenever I am feeling sorry for myself. But unless I have done something to change my mood then when that craving fades it is perfectly likely that I will still be feeling down, so a new craving will be launched as soon as the first one fades. This is enormously difficult to manage because if I do nothing to change how I feel then the cravings will keep coming and drawing down my resolve. But not only are emotional cravings likely to keep coming they are also going to be very powerful and this is due to a general property of how brains work.

Information is remembered more strongly if it is accompanied by strong emotion. It does this because if there was strong emotion present at the same time as a particular event occurred then this means that the incident was important in some way. So it is important that this be remembered firmly. Emotional triggers, by their nature, are always accompanied by emotion, so they are remembered forcefully. This means that their response; a craving, will also be powerful.

There are two general routes into addiction for those that are susceptible. One way is to start drinking and then the slowly strengthening triggers cause us to drink more and more. This brings on the emotional changes caused by alcohol-tolerance and these lock our addiction into place. The other path is that some persistent distress or severe trauma causes us to drink for relief over an extended period. The pursuit of relief encourages us to drink and this causes our drinking triggers to strengthen. Then alcohol-tolerance sets in and this traps us into drinking to relieve the symptoms that are themselves now also *caused* by drinking. If at this point the original distress is removed then we still drink because we are trapped by the emotional consequences of long-term drinking. But this only happens to those that are susceptible to addiction; it does not happen to normal drinkers. This point has been made before but it needs repeating in the context of emotional triggers. If a normal drinker suffers some distress over an extended period then they strengthen drinking triggers and bring on alcohol-tolerance in exactly the same way that we do. But at the same time as they strengthen drinking triggers they also strengthen alcohol-avoiding triggers and this makes them behave quite differently if the distress ceases. Firstly the alcohol-avoiding triggers will sometimes steer them away from drinking excessively (thus strengthening alcohol-avoiding triggers instead of drinking triggers) and this keeps their drinking somewhat moderated. But also, if the cause of the original distress is removed then they have those alcohol-avoiding triggers that will spontaneously return their drinking to a regulated level. We do not have that. We do not have effective alcohol-avoiding triggers, so regardless of whether we drank while we were younger and this strengthened over time, or we drank to escape some significant distress or trauma, then the consequence is the same: the triggers of our reward system begin to strengthen without limit and then the emotional changes of alcohol-tolerance lock addiction into place.

If our route into addiction was that we were drinking to gain relief from some trauma then counselling that eases this trauma may remove some of that distress but it does not make us able to drink normally again. Yes, it will lift that particular pain from our lives, but it does not create the ability to form alcohol-avoiding triggers, and it does not remove the triggers that have formed, so we remain captured by addiction. If this was the route into addiction then there are two distinct issues to address; the trauma *and* the addiction. Addiction cannot be overcome while the pain of the trauma remains because that distress makes relapse almost inevitable. There are two issues and both need to be addressed because one cannot be relieved while the other remains. But psychological trauma is not the only source of persistent distress. While I drank I did terrible things; things that brought enormous shame and guilt on myself, and things that hurt others. I may have done these because my judgement was compromised by alcohol but I still did them and I can't ignore this because the shame, guilt, and remorse caused by these all fire drinking triggers when I dwell on them. It is essential that I do whatever I can to relieve the burden of the guilt and shame that I carry and that I take steps to mitigate any trauma I have suffered at the hands of others, because failing to do so ensures that adverse emotions will persist. If left to run their course then these will slowly corrode my resolve and this invites relapse.

All negative emotions bring on cravings, and resisting cravings drains resolve, so I need to do what I can to reduce that burden. I can apply some of the same remedies for cravings caused by emotional triggers that I use for regular cravings and these are; describe, delay, distract and deny, but there is more I can do for these specific triggers. Distraction will help but I can make this more effective if the distracting activity is one that ends by lifting my mood. Activities that leave me with a sense of accomplishment, or that I've done something worthwhile, will displace the emotion that caused the problem and this means that I won't re-trigger myself when the task is complete. So it is well worth identifying a list of jobs, projects or tasks that will do this and it is also worth taking the time to have everything ready to be able to start them at a moment's notice. But for each adverse emotion there are also specific actions I can take to mitigate them. There are whole books, courses and groups devoted to improving our enjoyment of life, and many of these will help in a general way. But here are some simple ways to deal with these emotions specifically in relation to alcoholism.

Feeling Down: If I am feeling; miserable, sorry for myself, trapped, lonely or lost then I need to lift my spirits and the simplest fix is to do something that makes me feel good. The things that make us feel good vary enormously from person to person but here are some ideas to indicate the variety of fast and accessible ways to turn things around: take a long bath, enjoy a scenic view, have a food treat (sweets, savouries, a special meal), play some uplifting music loud and dance to it, or watch a favourite happy movie or engaging programme. What helped me was having a list of these because the times that I needed to do something were also the times that I was least able to come up with ideas about what it was I should do.

The opposite of feeling sorry for myself is feeling grateful for what I have and I can use this to help myself too. If I catch myself feeling down then mentally listing thing I am grateful for will turn the mood. If I imagine losing the things I am lucky to have then I will appreciated them better. I don't even need to be too successful in this as the mere act of thinking about what I am grateful for will help. I can narrow the task down even further by listing just the things I am grateful for since I stopped drinking, and that list is long. It is also important to remember the things that I *don't* have since stopping drinking because some of the biggest benefits I got were not what I gained but what I lost. For example I no longer come to in the shower remembering bits of what I did the night before and panicking about what I can't recall. I don't have the hangovers to push though for hours and I don't worry about how much I spent. I don't have to keep lists of who I need to avoid or how I am going to explain myself to them, and I don't start the day fretting about how I get my next drink; when, where, what and with whom. There is a lot I'm grateful to have lost and searching out some of these will often break me out of a spell of "poor me!"

Frustration: We get frustrated when we are unable to change or achieve something that we want to, and the key word that helps me here is "unable" because frustration comes from absence of control. Frustration is a self-imposed pain. Nothing is gained from it and my distress achieves nothing because the object of the frustration remains unchanged. There is a very simple way to fix this but as with so many things in recovery simple is not the same as easy. To remove the frustration from an event what I have to do is work out if I can change it or if I can't. If I *can* change it then I need to *do something* to make it change, if I *can't* change it then I must *accept* it, and that's it! If I can't immediately change something then I must accept it or I bring pointless frustration on myself and that frustration will trigger cravings. Acceptance removes frustration but it takes practise to achieve because it isn't straightforward. First I have to successfully identify that I have no control over a problem and then I have to move that problem into acceptance. I have to acknowledge that "it is what it is" and wishing and wanting it different won't make it so no matter how long or how hard I try. I have to let it go.

Anxiety: Anxiety is a feeling of fear or apprehension about what is to come. I guess and double-guess what the future will bring but this is pointless. There's a Chinese proverb that says "When men talk of the future, the Gods laugh". The truth about the future is that my ability to predict it is spectacularly poor, yet I still do it and I make myself suffer by doing so. The remedy for anxiety is to bring my mind back to the present. There are many tricks we can use to do this and a simple one is this. Find a clock; note the time, the day of the week and the date. Then say out loud the time, day and date and ask yourself "What *should* I be doing right now? What *should* I be thinking about right now?" Whatever answer comes back then go and do that immediately. Another simple way to reduce one cause of anxiety is to adjust how I prioritise my time. If I do the things that I *should* do before the things that I *want* to do then this improves the satisfaction that I get from the day and this steadily reduces the nagging stress I get from knowing that I still have tasks outstanding.

Anger: My brain pays more attention to information that is associated with emotions and anger is the most potent of them all. This makes the cravings that are linked to anger extremely powerful, but they are also brief. The best thing I can do with a craving brought on by anger is to buy myself some time. I try to do something immediately; walk away, walk in the opposite direction from any alcohol source, and cool off. I try to do *anything* to avoid drinking in the immediate aftermath of getting angry and I tell myself that I don't have to resist this for long because I will calm down and will soon regain control. What I need is time, and what I need is for there to be no opportunity to drink until I have recovered my composure. Do *anything* that moves you away from alcohol for 30 minutes.

Guilt, Regret and Remorse: In exactly the same way that anxiety is brought on by speculating on the future, guilt, regret and remorse are brought on by dwelling on the past. The remedy for this is the same as for anxiety: bring myself back to thinking about the present... "What should I be doing right now? What should I be thinking about right now?" My mind is an avid time-traveller but I don't help myself when I do this and I had to learn to actively direct myself back to the present. This line helped me identify when I needed to pull my mind away from dwelling on the past: "It is OK to look at the past, but don't stare".

As with so many things in recovery knowing what to do and actually doing it are very different things and the discipline of bringing myself back to the present is a good example of this. When I did this well then I wasn't troubled by my past or afraid of the future. But we only notice a pain when it is present, not when it is absent. So when I constantly brought myself back to the present then the whole purpose of doing so ceased to be apparent. This is why it is so important to *keep doing what's working*. It is when I stop doing the things that keep me well that I begin to struggle. These disciplines help, but they only help if I keep doing them.

Fear of missing out (FOMO): Something I needed to challenge vigorously when I had a bout of FOMO is whether or not it was real. My memory deceives me terribly about alcohol by insisting that drinking was good when in fact it was often the very opposite, and this memory "drinking is fun" was projected into my expectations of the occasions that I wasn't even at. The big thing to determine was if I was missing out on fun, or I was missing out on drinking, because they are not the same thing even if my mind tries to tell me that they are. There is a simple way to find out. If I find myself thinking I am missing out on fun then I picture the 'fun' scene in my mind. There are always two elements in it: people and alcohol, but which am I drawn to? Next I reimagine the scene except I remove all the alcohol. I swap all the glasses of beer and wine with fruit juice and lemonade and test my reaction.

Very often my interest in the scene evaporates once there is no alcohol present. This shows me that I didn't think I was missing out on fun at all, what I was being drawn to was the alcohol. This method works well for things that are happening now and also for events in the future. I can use it to test my true feelings about events that are yet to come and are giving me FOMO. If I find that the scene no longer commands my interest once the alcohol is removed then it is not the people enjoying themselves that I am missing out on, it is the alcohol. However, if I find I *am* still drawn to the occasion then I don't need to hold back. If it is truly the occasion that I am drawn to then I can still go, but I can take some sensible precautions; have a way to leave if I need to, take my own alcohol-free drinks, and be accompanied by someone who knows that I'm not drinking. But if I found that that the scene wasn't interesting once the alcohol has been removed then I knew I wasn't missing out on anything worthwhile at all; I only wanted to go there because of the alcohol. In that case what I am missing out on is the chance to upset my friends or colleagues, do stupid things, embarrass myself, or do things I will regret. My life is improved *without* all of these so I am not missing out at all by not going; I am gaining.

I can also look at whether or not I am the cause of my own FOMO. Was I turning down social invitations that posed no risk of drinking? Often I did. For years I had only ever attended social occasions where drinking was involved and if I am honest about this then on many occasions alcohol was the main reason that I went. Once I stopped drinking I found that I had a fear of meeting groups of people because it was so long since I socialised sober that I wasn't certain that I could still do it. I found that I was turning down invitations to events and social occasions because of this fear and I had to confront this directly. I had to re-join the world. If I was invited to go to some sort of gathering but was being held back by this fear then I developed the practise of replying "yes" immediately and dealing with the fear later rather than dithering or declining. After forcing myself to go to social occasions a few times my confidence started to return and once I was at an event then it usually flowed along easily enough after I got past my initial apprehension. But one thing was very different about these occasions. What I found was that once I stopped drinking then I was no longer the last person to leave a party, often I was among the first. But I mostly found that being around drunk or partly drunk people is incredibly irritating and I often had to leave for that very reason. I still do.

There is one sense in which I *was* actually missing out and that is I no longer got the frequent but artificial emotional lift I got from alcohol. For years my mood had been chemically altered by alcohol and I needed to deliberately fill this gap or FOMO would fill it for me. I deliberately did something every day to put some joy into my life. I set aside a little time each day to do something that was just for me and this ensured that I always had something to look forward to. It didn't have to be anything large, I only needed it to be a bright spot in the day, and with a little thought and preparation I could arrange this easily enough. Another thing I learned to do was to seek out new experiences and give them a try. If they didn't turn out to be my thing then nothing was lost. People don't die wishing they'd done less in their lives; they die regretting the things they did not do. Whenever I felt down I had to remind myself that boredom is a choice, and so is loneliness. I had control over both of these and I needed to make better choices because either was certain to bring on a bout of FOMO.

Shame: We evolved to live in communities and a part of that evolution is that we adopt the standards and behaviours of the community. We aid our survival by being in a group, so we serve the aspirations of the group as well as our own and this is how we win the support of the group. The way we evolved to make our behaviour to conform to that of the group is that our mind punishes us if we fail to meet the group's standards. This punishment is delivered in the form of shame. I feel shame when my behaviour is not aligned to that of my community, and my drinking definitely did not meet that standard. But I don't only impose shame on myself; I feel it from others too. Public opinion doesn't usually make a factual judgement about alcoholism, it makes a moral one. Normal drinkers have a completely different daily experience to us when it comes to alcohol. They do not have an out-of-control reward system, they are motivated away from alcohol when drinking is unwise, their memories are not hopelessly biased in favour of alcohol, their mood hasn't changed in response to frequent drinking, and their ability to freely choose if they should drink or not drink is intact. All of this has a direct bearing on how people judged me because praise and shame are only applied to actions that are freely willed. Only actions that are freely chosen are seen as deserving of credit or blame and this is where people draw an incorrect conclusion. Normal drinkers expect that I have the same free-will regarding alcohol as they do, so they assumed that I had *chosen* this course of action and was therefore deserving of condemnation. They don't do this out of malice. They make this judgement based on their own experience not knowing that mine is radically different. The consequence of this accusation for me is shame, and this hurts terribly so I began to change my behaviour to avoid this pain.

The emotional discomfort of shame evolved to encourage us to change our behaviour to conform to that of the group, but when it came to my drinking I could not. I couldn't stop drinking but the shame it brought was painful, so I found ways to get around the problem. If no single person ever saw the full extent of my drinking then my drinking could *appear* to fall within acceptable norms, and I adjusted my behaviour to create this impression. I drank somewhere and then moved onto somewhere else for more, I drank in different places on different days, I bought alcohol in different places on different days, I lied about where I went, when, and for how long, I disposed of my empties discretely, and I hid alcohol and drank it un-seen. I hid alcohol and drank secretly because when I did this then nobody saw how much I drank and therefore I wasn't shamed for it. This hiding behaviour is not caused by alcohol, it is driven by shame. Experiencing shame is a drinking trigger in itself and bizarrely one part of my brain compels me to drink while another part punishes me for doing so. I needed to remove this shame and one of the most powerful things I could do was to learn that alcoholism was *not* something I had chosen or brought upon myself. Much of that has already been explained but there is more. Not only is alcoholism not chosen, it is also not rare. In fact it is far more common than most people expect. I felt shame because I did not conform to a standard that society expects when it comes to drinking. But I can change the groups that I consider myself to be a member of. People in recovery communities have precisely the same issues and aspirations as I do, so in those communities I am not different, I am the norm. This means that I do not experience shame within these communities. If we want to unburden ourselves of shame then we need to find and routinely engage in some sort of recovery community. Do it, because despite your apprehension you will not be judged. A recovery community is the one place I cannot be judged for my drinking, and I cannot be judged within this group because my behaviour is the norm, not the exception.

This chapter has listed ways to address some specific emotions in relation to drinking but there are also some things that will help regardless of the feeling. All emotions are the products of either what my senses are discovering or the thoughts occupying my mind. The parts of my brain that generate emotion can't distinguish between what is happening and what is imagined. It generates the appropriate emotion for the circumstances regardless of whether it is real or imaginary. The more I allow my thoughts to wander and speculate then the more often I create emotions that are unrelated to my immediate circumstances. But once I stopped drinking then my emotions were no longer dulled or muted by alcohol, they came into a racing mind and were raw and vivid. Their impact could be shocking and the cravings they launched were powerful but what I most needed to *not* do was simply sit there and wait for them to go away. "It will pass" is poor advice for these occasions. The better advice is to *do something* to make it pass. If I sit with the emotion then this brings in more and more related thoughts and these will intensify it, make it continue longer, and keep re-triggering me. I make the craving period last longer because allowing negative emotions to persist causes cravings to recur exactly as though I was sitting in a bar full of alcohol and people drinking. What I need to do is identify the emotion and then do something to negate it. When I do this then I stop re-firing the trigger that is causing the cravings to persist.

Vigorous exercise is a good circuit-breaker for an adverse mood. This goes beyond just going for a stroll, it means getting my heart-rate up for a while and the benefit I get from this is endorphins. Endorphins are some of the brain's own feel-good chemicals and these are released after significant exertion, so I can deliberately use this to my advantage. If I am feeling down then one option is take some sharp exercise. This will outlast the craving and at the end of it my mood will be lifted so I won't be immediately re-triggered.

Another universal way to deal with emotions that are pulling me down is to talk to someone. When I engage in conversation then my mind has to work hard to analyse the other person's words and to prepare a response. What conversation does is it forces my mind to change the subject and when I start thinking about something different then the original emotion is stopped. The best people to talk to when I find myself in this position are other people in recovery because they understand the importance of this need to talk and they will deliberately help the conversation move along.

Regardless of the emotion one of the simplest things I can do to dislodge it is to name it. I identify it and say its name out loud. If I am feeling the need to drink *and* I am feeling miserable, angry, frustrated, embarrassed, guilty or ashamed, then this is the trigger. When I identify it and explain it to myself then I steer my attention to the cause of the problem instead of wallowing in it, and when I know the specific cause then I can apply the specific remedy. Even thinking about the action I should take will help and my mind will explore this automatically once it is prompted where to look.

I can reduce how often I get triggered by emotions by keeping my thoughts in the present and focussing on what is happening around me, right now, right where I am. Idle time is my enemy because when my brain has spare processing capacity then unresolved issues and problems from my past are brought forward for further consideration, and these spin up unwanted emotions. This is guaranteed to happen when I have time alone with my thoughts. But I can do a lot better than simply responding to these emotion-related cravings as they come. I can anticipate certain times when these emotions *will* come, and I can proactively work to prevent or minimise them.

I know that time alone will be challenging so I can make deliberate plans to fill as much of that time as possible with *doing* something. The other times I most urgently need to fill are the times that I used to routinely drink, and I know when these are. The best sorts of activity for these times are those that involve other people, those that leave me with a sense of achievement or worthiness, and those that require my full concentration. I also need to give my day a highlight or I will get the feeling that I am missing out by not drinking and then become dissatisfied with my sobriety. There are things I can deliberately *do* to reduce triggering myself with negative emotions and there are also things I can deliberately avoid. In particular there are some things I should avoid dwelling on because they are *guaranteed* to be problematic; dwelling on the past will make me miserable, dwelling on the future will make me anxious, dwelling on the bad things I have done will bring on remorse, dwelling on people I have hurt will bring on guilt, and dwelling on bad things that people have done to me will bring on resentment. In the short-term we need to minimise the time we spend thinking about these but later on we need to address them. In a later chapter we will look at how to stop all of these things from troubling us because that undercurrent of distress destroys resolve and can lead to relapse, but early on I needed to stop them from pulling me down. There were five things on that list; the past, the future, bad things I've done, people I've hurt, and things people have done that hurt me. I needed to limit the damage that each of these did until I got around to removing the pain from them, and the temporary measure was to do this: - I made a list, under each of those headings, of the things that were distressing to think about. The lists weren't huge but some of the items in them had a big impact on how I felt if I allowed myself to dwell on them. These lists told me where to *not* look. What I had to do is notice when I was thinking about one of the items on the list and deliberately change my line of thought. I needed to change the subject and the sooner the better, otherwise fear, anxiety, and depression were going to settle in. When I caught myself thinking about one of the listed items then I needed change the subject. I forced myself to think about something else with "What should I be doing right now? What should I be thinking about right now?" This is a difficult discipline to master and I certainly didn't get it right every time, but I got better at it with practise and it helped me by removing a background rumble of unnecessary distress and the cravings they triggered.

As time passed then more and more of my drinking triggers had their vigour stripped away and I no longer had to constantly fight off the demands that I drink. It took a while but as long as I didn't drink in response to a craving then this was guaranteed to happen. And for as long as I didn't drink then my mind would calm down and my mood and inner sense of well-being improved; this too was guaranteed. What I most needed was to be able to do is to stay the course and allow this all to happen. But the challenge isn't simple because we simultaneously fight on five different fronts: cravings, resolve, self-sabotaging thoughts, false memory, and adverse emotions. This book has identified a simple plan for dealing with each of these. This chapter identified the key emotions of addiction, why they are problematic, and what to do about them. But as time progressed and the intensity of the cravings fell away then these emotions climbed in significance. I slowly learned that the real challenge wasn't to stop drinking, but to stay stopped, and that emotions were the key to this.

Abstinence and Recovery

Abstinence and recovery are two completely different things. Abstinence is stopping the consumption of alcohol whereas recovery is achieving a state of well-being wherein the *desire* to drink no longer arises. Recovery is not possible while I am still drinking so the first step is to stop that, but stopping drinking only gets me so far. It does not prevent me from wanting to drink at some point in the future. The enduring challenge here is the single piece of self-sabotage "a drink will make you feel better" and this is so persuasive because it is true... it will. The objective in recovery is to achieve the mental state whereby that particular piece of self-sabotage either never occurs, or when it does it is unconvincing. Recovery is about achieving an emotional contentment that doesn't require alcohol to "improve" it. Stopping drinking is not recovery; it is a precursor to recovery. Abstinence and recovery are nothing like as closely linked as I expected because stopping drinking on its own does not advance recovery at all.

If, at the height of my drinking I had been castaway on a tropical island where there was plenty of food, shelter and water but no alcohol, then for the length of that stay I would be abstinent. If I was rescued after a year then I would have a sobriety "day count" of 365, but how recovered would I be? Well that would be none. If I was rescued after not drinking for a whole year then I would have gone and got completely, rotten drunk at the very first opportunity. The score line would be: Abstinence - 365: Recovery - 0. Stopping drinking does not automatically advance recovery and I have to work at recovery just like I have to work at abstinence.

Stopping drinking isn't the entirety of the challenge and if I thought that it was then I'd be setting myself up for a fall because abstinence and recovery have entirely different objectives. Abstinence requires continuous sobriety whereas recovery requires emotional wellness. This is what prevents "a drink will make me feel better" and the other self-sabotage from prevailing. Abstinence and recovery each has its own challenges and each has its own tools for addressing those challenges. The second cannot begin without the former, but as the challenge of stopping drinking recedes then the importance of staying stopped, recovery, rises. It isn't that I step from one course of action to another; it is that one set of tools becomes less frequently needed and another set becomes increasingly significant. The challenge changes over time and I must change with it because I cannot rely on my sober-days count to keep me safe. In reality that count gives me no protection whatsoever because it is what I do each day that either keeps me well or sees me drink again.

The timeline of recovery varies enormously from person to person. The physical recovery of our brain and body is guaranteed to happen in the absence of alcohol but this happens at our body's own pace and each of us re-adapts at our own speed. There is no miracle moment in recovery that marks the end, indeed there is no end because there are some things I need to do, and some things to not do, for the rest of my life. Recovery from addiction is a direction rather than a destination and there are some disciplines I need to maintain forever if I am to keep myself well. With practice they become simple to follow and require little from me on a daily basis. But while there is no end to recovery there *are* some clearly noticeable progress markers along the way.

One of the first signs we get that our body is correcting itself after years of being adjusted for drinking is that sleep returns. This usually happens at around two or three weeks after our last drink and is quite marked when it arrives. Not only do we suddenly get to sleep again but the sleep is different: it leaves us refreshed and bright in a way that we aren't accustomed to. While the first big change that *we* notice from stopping drinking is that sleep returns, there are changes that other people see that we may not. Alcohol-tolerance causes us to operate with a heightened heart rate for an extended period, but it is quite specific in the way that this happens. Our mind and body are prepared as though there is some imminent danger that we need to be ready to react to. Our heart rate is accelerated and blood is diverted from the skin to our large muscles, and this is the cause of our pale complexion. When we stop drinking then these precautions are stepped down and while we may not see them, others do: people start to comment that we are looking well. What they have noticed is that colour has returned to our skin. But there are two other less obvious changes and they are that we stand taller, and our mood brightens.

As the days since my last drink mounted up then my sense of hopelessness started to fade and my self-image lifted. I no longer felt the depth of worthlessness that I did and this is what caused the change in my posture and improvement in my mood. When colour returns to our complexion then good sleep is not far away because the elevated heart rate, alertness and the inability to sleep are all parts of the same process. While I drank my brain tried to keep me awake so that I could respond to danger but when that need disappeared then it relaxed and I experienced sleep that was unfamiliar: it was deep, satisfying and refreshing. Refreshing sleep is one of the great rewards of stopping drinking that is easily overlooked.

Alcohol-tolerance changes the release rates of several key chemicals and in the prolonged absence of alcohol each of these re-adjusts to find a new normal. Each of these chemicals has multiple roles in the brain or body and when they all adjust at the same time then this causes some chaotic outcomes: our mood can be all over the place. Getting sober is a wild ride for our emotions and they leap from one extreme to another at the slightest prompting. We feel this so strongly because we aren't used to emotions coming quite like this. For years we have smothered our emotions with alcohol but now we feel them and they come through incredibly vividly. This isn't a bad thing; this is how they are supposed to be, it showed me that I was getting better and that my brain and body were recovering. So when you experience them then acknowledge this. Emotional volatility isn't something terrible that is happening it is us recovering our proper emotions. It is a part of the healing that is happening.

There is one notable experience in this process that happens to many people and this is often referred to as the "Pink Cloud". As all the chemicals of addiction readjust their release rates then this inevitably affects our mood. Lowered serotonin and endorphin release rates caused us to be depressed and withdrawn while we weren't drunk but they now seek new levels and for some people these head towards their optimal position and then overshoot the mark. For a while we can have an oversupply of serotonin and endorphins and this leaves us with a feeling that all is well in the world. We are cheerful and bright, and although we are still confronted by frequent and intense cravings the rewards of sobriety seems to far outweigh the difficulty of carrying on. Unfortunately the Pink Cloud doesn't last forever and coming down from it we can start to feel the opposite. It can seem that the hard work no longer brings the rewards that it used to.

By the time I got to a month or so since my last drink then things were noticeably different. I still got very frequent cravings and they were still strong but they weren't as strong as they were, and if I compared them to what that first week was like then I could see this change. But more noticeable than the decline in craving intensity was that most of consequences of alcohol-tolerance were fading. The worst of the anxiety had gone, sleep had returned, and while I still had a racing mind this too was calming down.

Once the defensive measures of alcohol-tolerance started to dissipate then I felt a lot different within myself and this in itself presented a whole new challenge. It should be that after a month or so, when the cravings are smaller and my mood had lifted markedly, that I was far more able to carry on and stay alcohol-free. But this was not the case. It didn't get easier; it changed. The challenge shifted from fighting off cravings to managing my resolve and the self-sabotaging ideas. I needed to steadily work at maintaining my resolve while at the same time it no longer seemed necessary to do so. This step change was a tricky one to negotiate. I have no direct means of knowing the state of my resolve but I needed to keep it boosted up regardless. This was difficult to achieve when there seemed to be no need to do so but frequent contact with a recovery community kept this 'front and centre' for me.

Initially my sole challenge was to overcome the massive urges to drink during withdrawal. Then it was to stay off alcohol until the cravings dropped in intensity enough for me to get through my days without needing to fight them off every moment. These two are parts of abstinence, and once I was past them I didn't re-tread those paths. The long-term actions are those related to my emotional triggers.

The unpredictability of the world guarantees that powerful emotional triggers will sometimes be fired for the rest of my life, and I have to learn to negotiate this. If my resolve is in good shape then I can get past sudden difficult events without too much difficulty, in fact my sobriety becomes an asset at these times. But if I experience persistent distress then this will steadily corrode my resolve until "a drink will make you feel better" sounds too attractive to resist. There are several things I can do about this. I can continue to work to keep my resolve high, I can deliberately act to improve my day to day emotional state, and I can remove many sources of enduring distress. If I do all of these then I will experience fewer cravings and this in turn will reduce the flow of self-sabotaging thoughts. When I do this successfully then I not only make myself happier I also remove the very things that are most likely to cause relapse, because when I am content in my recovery then the need to drink simply doesn't occur. Every time I improve the way we feel about myself and my place in the world I get a twofold gain; I feel happier, and I deny self-sabotage the opportunity to establish itself and grow.

If I am to achieve an enduring sobriety then I must work at my emotional wellness from both ends. I need to remove things from my life that cause me enduring distress and I need to enhance or insert things into my life that increase contentment. I aim towards achieving a state where having a drink never appears to offer me any advantage, because if I do this then the self-sabotaging thoughts become completely powerless. This is the challenge of recovery and staying stopped.

Recovery isn't about the pursuit of some magical nirvana. For the most part the contentment I seek is what is left behind if I get rid of the unwanted baggage in my mind and concentrate on living today rather than in the past or the future. This direction change from fighting cravings to improving our mental well-being is a significant one but it is not something that suddenly happens. I didn't one day reach a point where I suddenly shifted my effort from preventing myself from picking up a drink to changing how I live. What happens is that one becomes less important over time while the significance of the other increases. Nevertheless I *must* manage my emotional state if I am to avoid relapse. Just as there are many moving parts in addiction there are many components in achieving this wellness, but essentially they fall into two parts; I need to clear up the past so that it no longer haunts me, and I have to live in ways that improve rather than depress my daily experience. Many people will neglect or choose to not attend to these but it places them at risk because it leaves a burden of distress in place that encourages self-sabotage and relapse. My life needs to be unshackled from the past if I am to be able to enjoy it freely, and when I am comfortable with my life then the need to drink does not recur. But this does not happen without effort. I need to *do* the things that will make this happen.

The Past

There are so many appalling things I did while I was drinking that my mind was strewn with the litter of chaos and destruction. There were terrible things I did, things I should have done but did not, opportunities lost, aspirations destroyed, and terrible harm done to others; all caused by my drinking. These things cannot be wished away or ignored. They happened, I was responsible for them, and they impose a heavy burden of shame and guilt that is enduring. They are direct consequences of my addiction and they do not magically disappear when I stop drinking; they leave a lingering toll.

Some incidents from my past keep coming into my mind and them they will not simply fade away because a specific function of my brain keeps calling them back. Our brain requires information to be orderly and resolved since lack of certainty causes indecisiveness and this can be disastrous when it comes to survival. So brains evolved to have a mechanism for trying to tidy up unsatisfactory information and we recognise that process as "worry". The brain uses idle time to review unresolved or incomplete information to see if it can be brought to a better conclusion, and this is what guarantees that unsatisfactory incidents from my past will keep coming back to haunt me. A simple example of it working is this. If, in conversation, I struggle to remember a particular detail; a name, a location, a detail or whatever, then it can suddenly pop into my mind hours or even days later. My mind uses idle time to process unresolved, incomplete or unsatisfactory information. Another feature of my brain ensures that this review will be uncomfortable, and this is caused by the way that our emotions are created.

Emotions are created in the subconscious part of our brain and that part of our brain evolved long before our higher, conscious, cognitive functions. These newer mental capabilities include self-awareness, imagination, and the concept of time: past, present and future. But my subconscious mind does not have these capabilities. To my subconscious mind everything is personal, everything is real, and everything is now, and my emotions are prepared on this basis. This means that if I replay an unsatisfactory incident from the past in my mind, and I can't stop this from happening, then my brain recreates emotions as though it is happening now. I get the same distress, anger, frustration, anxiety etc. as I did when the incident first occurred. The intensity of these emotions is a little lower, but they are the same emotions nonetheless. All of these emotions trigger cravings. This is why all the issues from my past leave an undercurrent of distress that pulls my mood down and initiates a constant flow of self-sabotaging ideas. If I can stop these thoughts from silently processing away in the background then I can remove a huge burden of effort from my recovery.

The way to take the distress out of issues in my past is to stop the ideas recurring, and the way to do that is to bring each of them to some sort of conclusion. While an issue remains unresolved then worry will bring it back into my mind and I will keep looping through it, time after time, forever. But if I can bring the issue to some kind of closure then this prevents it being brought back for further consideration, and the accompanying emotions, cravings and self-sabotaging ideas stop too. There are different ways to deal with unresolved issues and these divide the problem into three parts: - Things I have done that only hurt me, things I have done that hurt others, and things others have done that hurt me. I drew up three lists, one for each heading, of the things from my past that most troubled me. I wasn't looking for *all* of the bad thangs that I'd ever done or *all* the bad things that had ever happened to me, I only recorded the ones that as I recalled them gave me a bad emotional reaction. I listed the events that popped up both frequently *and* that made me squirm inside or get angry or frustrated when I thought of them. They weren't all necessarily directly related to my drinking. The events that caused me the biggest distress were the ones that I least wanted to acknowledge, but they were also the most important, so it took brutal honesty to make sure that I wasn't omitting to record the very things that were the most important to deal with. What I least wanted to record were the things that most urgently needed addressing. But I didn't need to record every single bad thing that ever happened. If it didn't keep coming back *and* it didn't hurt when I thought about it then there was no need to fix it.

Recording all the things that I needed to bring to a conclusion was hard to do and it was incredibly confronting. But the hardest part was to not leave off that list the things that most needed attention. The things I did not want to admit the most were the ones that were most important to deal with. The lists made appalling reading but there was one very important thing to note about them, and that was that they were not endless. The scale of the problem was finite. One by one I could bring each of these to closure, and every time I resolved an issue then it reduced the undertow of distress a little more.

Things I did that only hurt me:

This is the easiest group of issues to deal with and is related to the distress I put myself under when I hold secrets. Keeping secrets is intellectually demanding. My mind knows that each secret is an unsatisfactorily resolved issue, so it keeps bringing it back along with its associated emotions. But secrets have an additional emotion associated with them, and that is fear. Guilty secrets carry with them the fear that if they are exposed then shame will follow, and *that* is the burden that I can ease. The process is simple, but it is deeply uncomfortable to perform. My mind anticipates that I will be judged badly if the secret is exposed, that shame will follow, and this is the source of the fear. But if I tell my secrets and *do not* receive condemnation then the fear associated with that secret dissipates because shame *did not* follow. To remove the distress of a secret I simply have to tell it to someone that doesn't judge me for it. "All you have to do is to tell someone your secrets" is a very easy thing to say but it is incredibly uncomfortable to do. The trick is to find the right people and the right occasions to do this.

A person with whom I share these secrets has to be someone that will keep them confidential, but also someone that will hear them without passing judgement. This may seem a tall order but it is far easier than might be expected. Any rehab' or alcohol counselling will certainly do this in one way or another and I found that some of the people I had become comfortable with in the recovery community could also serve this purpose. I could use the informal periods at meetings to drop my secrets into conversations one by one or I could use a private conversation with someone I felt comfortable with to unload a bundle of them. I did both. It was desperately uncomfortable to do but the relief is real. This method of reducing distress by telling my secrets is not new or unique to recovery; it is a common practise around the world. Psychologists use it, it is a central tenet of both Buddhism and Catholicism, and it has been traditional wisdom for a long time, hence the expressions; "confession is good for the soul", to "get it off your chest" and "a problem shared is a problem halved". The extent to which this process is successful depends on finding the right person to hear the secrets and exposing them all. The secrets that most urgently needed to be exposed are the ones that cause the most distress and these are the very issues that are the most difficult to admit. But if a secret is withheld then so is relief from its burden. To be effective this task required completeness and that in turn requires brutal self-honesty. What I withheld would continue to hurt me and the burden of what I did not disclose would never go away. But it was hard to do.

Getting rid of all my secrets didn't have an instant uplifting effect, the benefit was felt differently. It was not a moment when the clouds parted and heavenly choirs sang, it was more like when a lingering pain ceased. I did not feel a sudden relief, other than that I had got past a very uncomfortable task. The relief was in the time that followed. Once this was done then I removed an undertow of anxiety from my life but it was a bit like not noticing the moment that a headache disappears. We don't feel it in that moment because we don't directly notice the benefit when something bad stops happening. But it was real and it was there. I got an overall lift in my mood when the continuous and nagging anxiety ended.

Things I did that hurt others:

The first list dealt with the enduring shame and fear that came from holding secrets and the second list addresses guilt and remorse. These events happened in the past but my mind kept bringing them back for consideration because they remained unresolved in one way or another, and in this respect they were still active. What I had to do with these was bring them to a clear conclusion and I can prevent these issues looping relentlessly in my mind by engineering an ending to them. I can't do the items in this list as a group, I have to attend to them one by one, and while I didn't need the help of an independent person to do this successfully, it was still enormously challenging. But again, like my secrets, the issues I most needed to address were the ones that recurred frequently *and* that caused me distress. I didn't need to deal with every bad thing I had ever done to anyone, only the ones that kept coming back into my mind and causing me distress.

I brought each issue in this list to a conclusion one by one and I did this directly with the person I had wronged. This is what makes the task so challenging but the relief gained is huge. There are many different ways that an outstanding wrong can be drawn to closure and here are the three commonest outcomes: - The person can demand something in compensation for the wrong, the person may never want to talk to me again, or, and this is the best possible result, I might be forgiven. Each of these three outcomes brings the matter to an end. If the matter is forgiven then there is nothing left to linger on, if they demanded some action in compensation then the matter is forgiven when I undertake that action, and if they never want to talk to me again then there's nothing further to be done that can ever change what has happened. In all three cases the issue has found an ending, and my mind will stop bringing it back as an issue to worry into conclusion because it now has one. This prevents the issue roaming around in my mind causing distress. It is easy to describe this process, but it was extremely uncomfortable to go on and do it.

What I do with each item on the list is to meet the person concerned (in person where this is possible) and raise the matter is such a way that it draws out a conclusion. The way to achieve this is *not* to simply apologise. This is insufficient and will not bring the ending that I need because the issue remains unclosed, and here is why. Suppose that I dropped someone's plate and it broke. If I apologise then does the plate put itself back together? No, it does not. The remedy is to offer to replace the person's plate with another, and then I might be forgiven. I need to do the equivalent of this with each of my issues. I arranged to meet, or at the very least talk with the person concerned, and I raised the matter directly. There are two sides to every issue but my concern was exclusively with resolving *my* part in it, not theirs. I talked about my actions that caused the problem, and I apologised without reservation for that; I should not have done that, I regret it terribly and I am sorry. I completely avoided mentioning their part in the problem, and I did not offer any justification or excuse, I just stuck to what I had done and nothing else. Then I asked this crucial question. "Is there anything I can do to put this right?" Their answer to this question is what allows me to bring this issue to a conclusion. If they say "OK, I did things too, let's leave it there"; then this is the best possible outcome. It is implicit forgiveness and the matter is concluded. Some say they never want to see or hear from me ever again, which is uncomfortable to hear, but this also concludes the matter because there is nothing I can ever do that will change the position. Or they might ask me to do something in compensation, and when I complete that then once again I am implicitly forgiven and the matter is ended.

These are enormously challenging confrontations to undertake but the rewards are huge in terms of removing recurring distress. As I completed each one I felt a sense of relief and that relief is enduring. In terms of timing I could not do this until my words had credibility. This meant I needed to have a significant run of sobriety before I attempted them otherwise my words could not be trusted... they'd heard it all before. But even if the timing is correct then there are still some circumstances that I must not attempt this closure kind of. There are circumstances where if I attempt to remove my own pain then it will cause distress for the other person, and I can't relieve my own distress simply by moving it to someone else. If I try this then it does not remove the problem, it only moves it to someone else, and that creates a new one. There are also times that we should not attempt such resolution and this occurs when it is hazardous or impossible do so. There aren't many occasions where this is the case but it does happen. For these occasions I needed to determine a suitable compensation and undertake that. This might be an activity that benefits the broader society rather than the specific individual. I need to define for myself an appropriate compensation for the harm I did and when I have performed that action then my due is repaid and the matter is concluded.

Making amends to others brings closure to my past mistakes and while it is incredibly difficult to do it is hugely beneficial. Even though I was reluctant to do this I had to force myself to do so, especially for the incidents that caused me the most distress. I did not do this only to relieve my own immediate suffering I did this to clear my path for staying stopped, because unaddressed and persistent distress leaves me anxious, erodes resolve, and ultimately invites relapse.

Things others did that hurt me:

The last list of issues to address is less confronting than the previous two for most people but extremely difficult for some. Events in my past where I have been badly treated by others leave me feeling angry and resentful and of all my emotional issues this is the most irrational. Holding a resentment does nothing at all to change the circumstances of the event and it does nothing at all to the person who caused me the injury. Holding a resentment is like taking poison yourself but expecting the other person to die. I achieve nothing by holding on to it but I persist nonetheless. The worry function of my brain keeps it circulating but resolution is never coming because the event is in the past and can't be changed. However, while I can't change the event I *can* change how I feel about the person and there are several ways to do this depending on the depth of the resentment.

The first thing to do is to test if I can't dismiss the resentment altogether. There are two sides to every story and I can look at what my part in this issue was. If I was partly to blame for what happened then why am I harbouring a grudge against the other person? If I can identify that I was responsible in part for what happened then the basis of the resentment collapses and many of them can be disposed of this way. For the resentments that remain I need to change how I view the person they concern.

I want other people to accept my flaws and forgive the mistakes I make. I get things wrong, I have done bad things, and a part of what I need to become well is the acceptance and forgiveness of others. Yet when it comes to resentments I apply a different standard: I do not forgive. Why do I expect other people to perform to a different standard than I hold myself to? It is an unreasonable position. I need to extend the same grace to other people that I want from them. I have no idea of the circumstances motivating the actions that hurt me, I barely understand my own, yet I am fast to judge them for it. I don't know what circumstances they are struggling with and I don't hold a monopoly on mental health difficulties. If I expect them to understand that I have challenges then I should acknowledge that they may have too. I need to shift my perception of how I see the individuals I hold resentments against and regard them not with anger but with compassion. When I allow them too to be flawed, and to make mistakes, then my frustration and anger dissipate. An apology would be nice but that is up to them not me. If they don't offer one then I shouldn't beat myself up for someone else's failings.

If this is insufficient to deflate a resentment then I use a less subtle approach: propaganda. It was mentioned earlier how self-sabotaging lies work like propaganda in that if we hear them often enough then we believe them to be true. We can use this same feature of how our brain works to deliberately change how we feel about a person we hold a resentment against. It isn't pretty, but it works. What I do is I write down a short paragraph wishing this person well: whatever I desire for myself I wish for them. It doesn't need to be a long passage, only two or three sentences, but it includes their name and what I wish for them. I then read this out loud to myself once every day for a month. At first it is hard to even speak the words without choking on them but as the days pass then my sentiment changes and I eventually end up meaning it. This may seem like a foolish exercise but it is not. At the end of the month the intense animosity I had for that person is gone.

These techniques will dramatically change or remove most resentments but there are some wrongs that we should not attempt to address like this. The incidence of alcoholism among those raised with childhood abuse is significantly higher than the norm and the same is true for people who have suffered sexual or domestic abuse. Traumatic events like this that cause deep and lasting suffering need to be dealt with in a focussed manner and not the generalised ways described here. They must not be ignored. We absolutely *must* do something to mitigate the distress due to severe trauma or we leave in place an issue that continues to cause persistent and severe pain and this will eventually collapse resolve. There are many community support groups to help those suffering the long term consequences of various types of abuse. They are places that will help people recover from this trauma and they are places to go without fear of shame or other consequences. They will help and there is no downside to them. If this is insufficient then professional help should be sought because the chance of achieving a long-term sobriety while still suppressing enduring suffering is small. Ultimately there is this truth. I need to forgive them, not because they deserve forgiveness, but because I deserve peace. We have to find ways to achieve this.

Dealing with my past has little to do with stopping drinking, but it has everything to do with staying stopped. Regardless of the sources of my distresses I need to do what I can to reduce them because persistent distress lowers resolve until the self-sabotaging lies sound convincing and I drink again. I cannot simply try to push these problems to the back of my mind because they will not stay there, worry will keep bringing them back. So, unpleasant as it may be, I have to take the steps to mitigate what I can. The result of doing this work is that I remove tier after tier of background discomfort from my mind and what is left behind is calm. But there is little point in going through these deeply uncomfortable processes if I only remove these distresses to have then replaced by new ones, so some changes in the way I live are in order to prevent this.

New Ways

The world is a chaotic place that is often grossly unfair. There will always be times when I am dissatisfied with life and upset by it and I have to work my way through these times just like everybody else. Stopping drinking doesn't make the world's problems stop, but it does restore my ability to do something about them. Many of life's stresses are unavoidable but I also bring a lot on myself that *can* be avoided. I can deliberately work to remove unnecessary distress from my life and this in turn will lower the amount of self-sabotaging chatter that I experience.

I didn't make any dramatic lifestyle changes initially, that was going to be too hard to sustain, what I did was engage some small disciplines that removed distress from my life. Each was a simple thing to do, each added more contentment to my day and on the days that I was content then the call to drink was entirely absent. None of these disciplines came easily, they all required effort to get underway, but once I'd started them they began to become almost automatic. They may seem trivial but these small changes help to bring contentment into my life and that peace avoids my addiction ever being triggered.

Do something about my problems. Over years of drinking I accumulated all manner of problems and some of them were big ones. Many of the difficulties in my life ceased to occur when I stopped drinking but others remained and I had to do something about them. But once again I am impeded by my characteristic to greatly favour now over later, because remedies that take a long time to achieve have little appeal to me. I am only poorly motivated to act to change something if the benefit of that action is a long way off. But this maxim told me what to do about issues like this: - "Advance towards the problem".

My accumulated problems appeared so large they seemed insurmountable but there is a feature of problem resolution that I can use to help myself, and it is this. I don't have to completely overcome a problem to gain significant relief from its burden; I only have to improve it. I only need to make progress on a problem for it to trouble me far less. I need to perform some action that moves me in the direction of resolving the problem because doing that first thing brings me huge relief.

When I am wrong then I apologise immediately. This may seem small but it can make a big difference. If I have done something wrong then I can either admit it or debate the point and try to talk my way around it. But if I delay an apology then the position worsens quite quickly. The other party starts to feel increasingly aggrieved, and I start to justify my own actions. As time passes the two positions polarise and it gets progressively harder to make an apology, and it becomes harder for the other person to accept it. But an immediate apology extinguishes the issue before it has a chance to escalate. It is uncomfortable admitting that I'm wrong but this course of action is the one that brings me significantly less grief in the longer term.

I don't need to be right all the time. I don't have to know everything, I don't always have to be right, and if someone is wrong then it is not necessary for me to correct them unless this improves the overall position. If the only purpose served by correcting someone is to demonstrate that they are wrong and that I am right then all I am doing is stroking my own ego, and it is big enough with that help. It is better not said as it will only make people dislike me. There are three test questions I can ask myself: Does it need saying? Does it need saying now? Does it need saying by me? Unless the answer to all three is "yes" then there is no gain in speaking out, only a penalty. On the other two points; knowing the answer, and being right, I don't need to do these. It is OK to not know the answer sometimes and it is OK to be mistaken. I do not know everything and I am not infallible. To pretend otherwise is not only being untrue to myself it is trying to deceive others. Both of these carries a burden of stress that is unnecessary and is easily avoided by honesty. So I speak honestly or I don't speak, any other course creates an avoidable distress.

I don't judge others. Our higher mental functions evolved after our subconscious mind, and emotions are the first language of the brain; they evolved long before speech. This causes an odd effect that, once I understood it, I could use to take a lot of distress from my life. Emotions are generated deep in my brain but my subconscious mind can't tell the difference between myself and other people, it doesn't distinguish between real and imagined, and it doesn't know about past or future. To my subconscious mind everything is real, everything is now, and everything is me. This means that if I say something insulting about someone else, or even just imagine it, then I experience emotion as though it was said to me and about me. If I look at something foolish that someone is doing and call it stupid then my emotional experience is as if I have just been called stupid. So if I find myself being judgemental of someone then I immediately think something good about them. This undoes the insult and replaces it with a compliment. My brain then creates the emotion as though *I* have just been praised and this replaces the insult. It takes practise to intercept the insult and reverse its effect but after a while I found that I started to make this correction automatically and this small adjustment takes a lot of moments of unnecessary anger and frustration out of my day.

Be deliberately social. While I was drinking I almost never went to any occasion that didn't involve alcohol and I usually drank beforehand to "get myself in the mood". I did this for years. It was a long time since I experienced a social event stone-cold sober and at first this was incredibly intimidating. But if I was to engage freely in the world again then I needed to become comfortable in social settings. I had to acknowledge that this was a problem and deliberately work at overcoming it. The first thing to do was to look at the fear; what is it that I was actually afraid of? Was I afraid of the risk of drinking? Was I afraid of not knowing how to speak to people? Was I afraid of not being the "life and soul" of the party? Was I afraid of having to explain why I wasn't drinking? Was I afraid that people wouldn't like me when I was sober? All of these fears were unfounded, irrational, or avoidable but I had to turn up to discover this.

If I go to an event at which I know there will be drinking there are simple things I can do to overcome the risk and these have already been mentioned; I can prepare a way to leave if I need to, I can identify and describe cravings as they come, I can take my own alcohol-free drinks if I am unsure of their availability, I can be accompanied by someone who knows I am not drinking, and I can move away from alcohol if I feel the need. Often these precautions gave me enough confidence to get through a triggering event but if I felt at risk of being overwhelmed then I always knew I could leave if I needed to.

The idea that people might not like me if I didn't drink and that I didn't live up to other peoples' expectations sober was simply ridiculous and the first gathering I attended without drinking showed me this. I do not become more interesting or more engaging when I drink; perhaps I thought I did but I was wrong. When people drink they start to talk rubbish, they get repetitive and generally become incredibly irritating. I was no different. I did not become more fun when I drank and I was fooling myself when I thought I did. So if I go to an occasion now I am not concerned that I won't perform up to expectations because I will exceed them. I should also not be concerned that I won't know what to say because what I say will now have merit, and anyway, if I don't know what to say then I don't have to talk and command attention, I can listen. I don't need to feel that it is my job to entertain, because it isn't. Nor am I required to stay the same just to please others. I am under no such obligation.

One of the things that troubled me a lot prior to an event was worrying about how I would explain to people why I was not drinking, but this involved a huge misconception on my part. I made the assumption that other people thought about alcohol the same way as I did; but they do not. I did not understand them and they did not understand me. I was preoccupied with thoughts of alcohol because for a long time alcohol was in my waking thoughts and with me throughout the day. But normal drinkers do not experience this. I am the one preoccupied by alcohol, not them, and they have no idea at all that alcohol commands so much of my attention as it does. It is only a big deal to me. They do not go to an occasion wondering if there will be enough to drink because it isn't that important to them. So if at an event someone says that they don't want a drink it isn't shocking. Maybe they are driving later, maybe they've had enough, or maybe they just don't feel like another. "No thank you" isn't an unusual response to being offered a drink, except to me. I sometimes prepared a good "excuse" for not drinking but the reality was that I rarely needed it because other people don't think it is unusual to *not* drink. Not only do many people not drink when they are at an occasion I also found it quite shocking to discover how little they drink when they do.

I overcame my fear of socialising by deliberately spending time with people and this is how I discovered that my fears were mostly unfounded. I would be nervous before going to an occasion but I usually discovered that it went just fine once I was there. The main fear is in the anticipation of the event rather than the event itself. I needed to push myself at first to get comfortable in social situations again and I had to show up for that confidence to return.

Stay in the present. There are many things that give me trouble if I dwell on them but poking around in the future will make me anxious and there are past events that cause me trouble if I look at them for too long. These have both been mentioned previously but bringing myself back to the present is something I have to do continuously and not just once or twice. There are many tricks we can use to pull ourselves away from an unwanted thought line and one has already been mentioned: "What should I be thinking about and what should I be doing right now?" Here is another: -

Choose something you aren't particularly familiar with from on your left side. Look at it, keep looking at it, and be curious about it for a couple of minutes. What is its purpose? Where did it come from? What is it made of? Where did those materials come from? Who put it together? How did it get here? Now repeat this with something chosen from on your right. Look at it and ask yourself questions about it. Then, while still looking at the item on your right imagine the item you chose on your left, and resume the questioning of that. After a couple of minutes swap the subjects around: look at the item to your left but imagine the item to your right and ask more curiosity questions about that. After a few minutes of this then the original thoughts that were consuming you will have been driven out because your brain doesn't have the capacity to keep that conversation going as well as thinking about and imagining other things. But regardless of the circumstances the easiest way to move my mind to the present is always to *do something*.

There are many ways to bring myself back to the here and now and many practises include it. Yoga, meditation, and mindfulness will all help with this and joining a local group that practises these will also help with our need to become socially comfortable again.

Expectations. I can't live entirely in the present. There are times when I need to explore the future to make prudent plans, but I often set myself up for disappointment when I do this. Yes, I need to make plans for some future event or project, but what I must avoid is visualising the success of its achievement. If I am thinking about some future event or project I am preparing for then I will do the planning but I never allow myself to daydream about its success, because this creates an expectation, and expectations are guaranteed to cause me frustration later on. When I dream up a picture of what I think *should* occur at some point in the future then I am always going to be disappointed because things don't happen as soon as I want, or as well as I want, and sometimes they don't happen at all. Expectations *always* create future disappointment and frustration. Fantasising about the future guarantees that I will be frustrated and the way to avoid this is to catch myself drifting away from the knowable and bring myself back to the known. It isn't an easy discipline to master but it is guaranteed to remove some distress from the future.

Control and frustration. There was a whole new discipline to learn when it came to control, change, and acceptance. As with many components of stopping drinking and recovery I needed to recognise a warning flag and then deliberately intervene with a specific action instead of letting my mind run its course. I needed to become sensitive to my level of frustration. I get frustrated when things aren't happening the way I want them to but most of the time this frustration is pointless because it achieves absolutely nothing; the situation remains unchanged. The discipline I needed to learn is to recognise mounting frustration and then test the circumstances causing it. Do I have direct and immediate control over this, or is control beyond my sphere of influence? Some simple examples of what I have no control over are; what other people think, do and say, what happens around me, and the outcomes of my efforts. Any or all of these can frustrate me but the frustration serves no purpose so I need to ask myself "am I being frustrated by something that I can control?" Very often I cannot; take traffic for example. If I am held up in rush-hour traffic then why allow frustration to build? All the other people in this traffic-jam haven't conspired together just to make me late;

they all have lives to live and they are delayed too. Frustration like this serves no purpose whatsoever yet and I spend much of my time becoming angry about things I can do nothing about. So I learned to sense the frustration rising, examine the source to see if I was trying to exercise control over something beyond my reach, and if so, let it go. If I *do* have control then I need to *do something* to alter the circumstances, but if I do not then I need to relax, breathe, accept that I can't change what is happening, and let it go past. I need to accept the things that I do not have immediate control over and let them flow past without disturbing me further. But this is far easier to say than to do. Some things I can push aside easily but sometimes they are more persistent.

Acceptance. The need to accept what is unchangeable has been mentioned in many places in this book, but what has not been described is how to do it. The more issues I can bring to acceptance then the more dissatisfaction I remove from my life and the more content I become. If I dwell on my problems then my mood goes dark and I become anxious, angry, fearful, resentful and depressed. The longer I dwell on these things then the more I intensify the emotion I am experiencing. For some things I need to recognise that what's done is done; there's nothing further that can be done to change the events so continuing to think on them will yield no benefit. I need to accept them for what they are and move on. But accepting things that I deeply want to be different is difficult. Some issues keep coming back into my mind for resolution but I never find it, so they keep coming back and going around and around. People say "get over it" and this is good advice, but it only tells me what to do, not how to do it. I needed to find ways to bring these problems to a conclusion so that they didn't keep coming back. The way to do this is to accept them for what they are, unchangeable, and to do this I have to find a way of looking at them that convinces me of their inevitability.

"Accept" is a verb and acceptance is an active process not a passive one. I can't just wait for acceptance to happen; I have to do something to make it happen. I need to consciously make a distinction about issues that are causing me anxiety: - Can I change this, or can't I? If I can't change this then I need to accept it and the trick here is in finding the key that allows me to change the way I perceive the problem. If a particular issue cannot be changed then it must be "accepted" for it to cease to cause me distress. This means I have to fully recognise that an issue can't be changed, e.g. it happened in the past and there's nothing to be done to change it, or it is happening now, or it will happen in the future and it is inevitable. I have to change the issue from "but it is wrong!" to "I don't like it, but I understand why it is so". When I achieve this then the issue will cease to be constantly brought back for resolution. My mind will accept that, unsatisfactory as it is, it is as resolved as it is ever going to be. This is done by inspecting each issue thoroughly and carefully. I keep looking at it until I am completely satisfied that there is nothing to be done to change it, *and* that I understand *why* I find it unsatisfactory.

The task is to bring each issue to a position where, when I reflect on it, it is emotionally neutral; this is the proof that something is truly accepted, and this is the outcome that I'm aiming for. To accept troublesome issues I need to concentrate on them and be undisturbed, so I do this quietly in my own space. I take time to fully immerse myself in each issue, one by one, and try to find the reasons why I am still holding onto them. This is identifying what it is that prevents me from accepting them. I have a list of reasons why I might accept something, and I test each issue against this list until I find a resolution.

- **I must accept this because I will never know the answer.** I will never know the answer to some questions. If I am never going to know the answer then continued searching is both endless and completely fruitless. Thinking further on this will never yield a solution... ever.

- **I must accept this even though it isn't fair.** Bad things happen. Bad things happen to everyone and nobody ever said that life was meant to be fair; it is not. The more I can recognize that life is inherently unfair then the easier it is to step past misfortune when it comes. I shouldn't hold onto something from the past because it isn't fair since something being unfair does not change the fact that it has happened. It is not going to magically change itself back again because it is unfair, so fair or not, it is done. "It's not fair" doesn't change anyone or anything, but it has a really bad effect on me. It makes me feel sorry for myself and nobody else is doing this, I am doing it to myself. I have to tell myself "it's not fair" one last time, then say "but life moves on".

- **I must accept this because I made a mistake.** I might try hard and aim high but I am not perfect. Nobody knows everything, nobody is always right, and nobody goes through life without making mistakes... nobody! If I expect constant perfection from myself then I have set an unachievable and invalid expectation. I do not have all the answers, it is OK to be wrong, and it is OK to make mistakes. People make mistakes and I am a person too. If I have made a mistake then I don't try to hide, minimise or justify it to myself because I won't be able to. I try not to repeat the mistake in the future, but I forgive myself for the ones I make. If an apology is in order or I need to make amends in some way then I do that. Otherwise I have to acknowledge the mistake, "I got that one completely wrong", and move on.

- **I must get over my pride and accept this.** Am I too proud to accept this? Do I look at this and think it's beneath me or not good enough for me? If so then the issue is not the real problem, it is my pride that is causing the trouble. I have to separate the facts from the feelings because on this occasion it is pride that is causing me the frustration; not someone else, or something else, but my own pride. I have to let it go.

- **I must accept this because people are not perfect.** Just as I make mistakes, so do other people. Other people aren't perfect, other people aren't always right, and other people make mistakes. When I allow other people to have failings instead of requiring them to be perfect then I am better able to accept their words and actions. People aren't perfect and that is a reality of life. Move on.

- **I must accept this because I have forgiven myself.** People are allowed to make mistakes. "To err is human". I am a person too. I want other people to forgive me so I have to extend that same grace to myself.

- **I must accept this because being in the right does not change it.** Believing that I am right achieves nothing whatsoever because the event remains unchanged. In the same way that being angry, remorseful, resentful or aggrieved achieves nothing, neither does this. The event does not change and I am simply inflicting suffering on myself for no purpose by thinking about this in terms of right and wrong. I have to get off my high horse, stop complaining about it, and move on; everyone else has.

- **I accept this because I have learned the lesson.** This makes the pain behind an issue meaningful. Sometimes bad things happen but this ends up being an important part of my personal growth. When I find the growth that I gained from the experience then I can move on.

- **I must accept this because I lack the means to change it.** This is about recognising the absence of control. Nothing will be different unless something changes, and if that change is beyond me then there is nothing whatsoever that I can do about it. If I cannot change it because I don't have the means to do so then thinking further on it will achieve nothing except keep me distressed. It is unchangeable. Let it go.

- **I must accept this because this is what has to happen.** This last one catches aspects of my life that I am unhappy about. Life isn't wonderful all the time and I often wish things were different, but they aren't. There may be some dissatisfaction with my current circumstances that I can't change, but the world is in constant flux and there will come a time that some things that are currently fixed *can* be changed. Sometimes I may need to endure what I am dissatisfied with while I undertake some lengthy process that will improve it. Either way, for the moment, I need to accept things as they are. A time may come that I can change this, but for the moment I cannot and therefore I must accept it or I just keep frustrating myself. It is what it is and this is what I must do because this is what has to happen.

Acceptance works like a salve, so if I find an explanation that closes an issue then I have to keep applying it. Things have a habit of un-accepting themselves so when they return I just re-apply the remedy because if I keep supplying the explanation for the issue then my mind will eventually stop bothering to bring it up. Ultimately acceptance hinges on this: I need to live in the world as it is, not as I want it to be. The more I can embrace this then the fewer issues will arise that I need to attend to. But I should not try to push all issues aside with acceptance, because some things cannot or should not be accepted. If something refuses to be accepted then I have to re-check the original premise, because acceptance may not be the correct remedy. My mind will only let me accept what *cannot* be changed. But if there is something I *can* do to change it then acceptance is never going to work. If I *can* change an issue then I must take some corrective action if I want relief from it. In particular, being accustomed to something unsatisfactory is no excuse for doing nothing about it. I should not continue making a mistake just because I've been making it for a long time. If I want relief from an issue then I need to change what can be changed regardless of how uncomfortable that might be.

Managing my self-esteem. How favourably I see the world is largely determined by how I feel within myself. We don't see things are *they* are, we see things as *we* are. But in the same way that I don't have an internal meter that tells me the state of my resolve I also don't have anything that directly lets me know how *I* am; but I can find out easily enough. The state of my self-esteem is mostly revealed by how I answer these four questions: - How loveable do I think I am? How valued do I think I am? How capable do I think am? and How worthy do I think I am?

These four combined give me an overall indication of how I feel about myself, and while I was still drinking my score for these was desperately low. But none of these are entirely fixed; there are things I can do to alter them.

How loveable do I think I am? As with many things in addiction the way to lift how loveable I feel is to work on the opposite end of the problem. Gifts do not make me more loved unless they are given unconditionally. But if I give gifts because I want to be forgiven or to be more loved then I do not give them freely, I attach conditions. This makes them not a gift, but a bribe, and I can't bribe people into loving me. The way to lift how loveable I feel is to address the opposite end of the problem and that is to stop doing the things that make me unlikeable. This is far easier than trying to make myself loveable and big gains can be won by small changes; do I interrupt or talk over people, do I take home worries to work, do I take work worries home, do I tell others how they should be living, do I listen to what others have to say, and so on. I can identify very many small things like this and they are easy to avoid with a little thought and application. When I stop doing unlikeable things then people like what's left behind, and so do I, because what is left behind is perfectly likeable.

Another way I can make myself feel more loveable is to address the personal characteristics that make me unlikeable. Changing my personal characteristics may seem like a big task but it isn't necessarily. I'm not trying to change myself wholesale; I just want to reduce the things that deter people from liking me, and the way to do this is switch emphasis and again work at the opposite end of the problem. I get a far better result by boosting the opposite characteristic than by trying to suppress a problematic one. For example, if pride is an issue then I concentrate on its opposite: humility. If I work at being more humble then this automatically reduces the prideful activity that others find unlikeable. Being humble does not make me less capable, but it does make me more likeable.

How valued do I think I am? I feel valued when people say "thank you" so the very easy way to feel more valued is to more often do the things that people will thank me for. I don't have to do big things to get gratitude, and all thanks count, so I do lots of little things. This needs no more of me than being thoughtful and considerate of others as I go through my days and it provides a simple source of thanks. All I have to do is be helpful. It was mentioned earlier that if I want my days to be more satisfying then I should do what I *should* do, before what I *want* to do, but I can improve on this. If I want to lift how valued I feel then I ask: - Is there something I should do for *someone else* before I do what I want to do for *myself*. And while I'm doing that I remember to thank others for what they do for me because when I thank someone then I improve *their* day and I get a lift from knowing I have done that.

How capable do I think am? This is an easy one to work on but it takes time and commitment. To improve how capable I feel I need to learn something new like a new skill, craft, ability, qualification, language etc. It is that simple. It doesn't matter what it is, or how large or how small, all I have to do is to learn something new.

How worthy do I think I am? If I spend my days doing things that I think are worthless then I will feel that I am worthless, so I need to have some significant activity in my life that makes me feel worthwhile.

There are some obvious things that I can do; I can redirect what was formerly drinking time towards my family, I can use that time to work on recovery, or I can throw myself into my work. Other things that make me feel worthy are activities that I can look at afterwards and say "that was worth doing". These could be projects or long-term activities that improve my own position but more powerful than any of these are activities that help other people or the community. Doing voluntary work that helps people (or animals) not only makes me feel worthy it is also likely to make me feel valued as sometimes I will be thanked for what I do. Community projects are a good opportunity to do this as this not only lifts my sense of worthiness it is an easy way to re-engage socially.

None of these actions described in this chapter are about stopping drinking they are all about *staying* stopped: recovery. Nothing and nobody else makes me drink again, only I can do that. When I am well within myself then apart from the faint murmur of remaining triggers the idea that I should drink again does not occur, or if it does then it is easily dismissed. However, if I become dissatisfied with my sober life then this sets the self-sabotage going, and this is what brings me down. I don't drink again after months or even years of being alcohol-free because I am driven to do so by the power of the cravings because they lack that power by then. I will drink again because my resolve is low, I feel low, and "a drink will make you feel better" becomes convincing. We don't drink again because the challenge is fierce; it is not. We drink again because our determination to stop has diminished and our self-sabotage does the rest. The two things required to keep me safe from this are maintaining my commitment to stopping and remaining emotionally well. The key skill to acquire is to become sensitive of my emotional condition, and then take corrective action is it is awry.

Emotional wellness is the prize we win for becoming alcohol-free and it is also our best defence, because when we are well then the biggest pieces of self-sabotage do not occur. For as long as we remain emotionally well then alcohol no longer presents itself as something attractive, in fact the opposite happens: when we are emotionally well then we reject any suggestion that we should drink as ridiculous. Maintaining our emotional well-being is the best defence against relapse... but despite our best intentions we aren't always successful.

Relapse

Stopping drinking is a monumental task. It requires that I recognise specific unwanted behaviour of my mind as it occurs and then contradict it. I have to do this with force of will while my condition wields dopamine which has the express purpose of directing my behaviour. That dopamine is supported by an unfaithful memory and sabotaging lies which constantly tell me that having a drink is a good idea. The challenge is not only a stern one but it continues without pause for weeks and months and only very slowly relaxes its grip.

It is amazing that anyone manages to overcome addiction yet most do, but nobody truly succeeds at their first attempt. Everyone that overcomes addiction fails before they succeed. My first failures were not being able to adhere to my own decisions about limiting how much I drank. I tried everything I could think of to control my drinking but I failed every time, and then I still tried and tried again. I was desperate to avoid the conclusion that I didn't want to believe; that I couldn't control my drinking and that I would have to stop completely. But eventually I could no longer deny the truth. My drinking was out of control and I could not regain control. It wasn't fun anymore, it was killing me. I couldn't stop, but I couldn't carry on either.

This was the pivotal point at which recovery became possible for me. It is the point at which denial collapsed and I realised that change wasn't simply something desirable, it was essential. This did not mean that I would be successful, what it meant was that it was no longer impossible. When I finally reached the point that the pain of carrying on drinking exceeded the pain of stopping then I gave it a try. But it was only when I first stopped drinking that I fully felt the extent to which I was captured by alcohol. In previous attempts I had lasted one, two or three days before drinking again but I had never before felt the full intensity of cravings nor the non-stop head chatter. It was a huge step to accept that I had to stop drinking, but it was an even bigger step to sustain that belief against an incessant barrage of massive cravings and self-sabotage. I wasn't prepared for the intensity of those cravings nor the extent to which my own mind would try to convince me to drink again. The research shows that very few are already sufficiently convinced of the necessity of their course to overcome these at their first attempt, and the great majority will drink again within a week. At first some will manage a few days, some will last a few weeks, and some fall into a prolonged pattern of stopping for a spell then drinking again. But, as a broad generalisation, with successive efforts we get better at recognising the challenges as they come, we get better at confronting them successfully, and we achieve longer stretches of sobriety.

If I manage to stop for a month or more then I not only weaken a lot of my drinking triggers but my brain undoes many of the changes it made to overcome alcohol-impairment and I feel far better within myself. If I *do* drink again however I immediately start re-strengthening my drinking triggers, and they recover their former vigour very quickly indeed.

We strengthen a drinking trigger when we drink in response to the craving it launches and we weaken the trigger when we don't. But the reward system evolved to accommodate changing circumstances and one way it does this is significant if I stop drinking for a period and then start again. This feature of the reward system is illustrated by how its triggers respond to a seasonal fruit in the wild. When I first meet a nutritious fruit then I take it, enjoy it, and establish a trigger. If the fruit remains available then each time I take some I am driven more strongly to seek it, and the trigger increases in strength for as long as that fruit remains available. But if I kept doing this when the fruit ceased to be in season then I would waste a lot of time and energy searching for fruit that would never be found. When the fruiting stops then the trigger to seek it out begins to fail, loses strength, and my interest in it reduces. But it is what the reward system does when that fruit comes back into season that is most important to us. When the fruit becomes available again then it would be inefficient to slowly bring that trigger back up to strength. If the fruit comes back into season then the most beneficial response is to restore that trigger to its full strength quickly, and this is precisely how the reward system behaves. The trigger for that fruit became weakened when the fruit was out of season, but it is still there. When fruit becomes available again then what remains of that trigger still motivates me somewhat to approach and take the fruit, and when I do then it is re-strengthened. But this time it isn't strengthened a little, it is strengthened *a lot*. If old triggers become re-activated then they assume their full former strength very quickly, and after only a few cycles of seeing and partaking of the fruit then that trigger is restored to its full prior strength. Triggers may lose their strength through repeated failure but they are never forgotten because they may become helpful again at some time in the future. They regain their former strength very quickly once they start to become successful again and unfortunately for us this is precisely what happens to all of our alcohol-related triggers. Drinking triggers may lose their strength through successive failure but they are not forgotten. We put huge effort into overcoming them and stripping their strength but we can never remove them completely. They sit there waiting to be reinvigorated, and if when we drink again then they recover their former strength alarmingly quickly.

Most people will not manage to remain entirely alcohol-free at their first attempt because the challenge posed by our self-sabotage is unfamiliar, severe and relentless. We may have made a conscious decision to stop but our mind still tries to persuade us to drink and we don't know how to deal with this conflict. One of the issues we face after a period of abstinence is that our mind begins to tell us that we have been successful and that we have beaten the problem. This is a deception but it is a seductive one. There are five changes that create this illusion; cravings lose their intensity, the effects of alcohol-tolerance reverse themselves out, the distance from despair means that we are no longer propelled by the need to escape our hopelessness, and Fading Affect Bias and our biased memory tell us that our drinking was a good thing. After a period without alcohol then we feel better within ourselves and we seem to be coping with the cravings we meet. This creates the illusion that maybe we can control it now, but we can't. The illusion is created by the challenge becoming less severe, not increased control on our part. Any attempt to return to drinking in a moderate way is guaranteed to fail sooner or later.

We might try drinking again within certain limits, like only on a Friday after work, but we cannot hold firm to this boundary. We may succeed in limiting our drinking like this for the first few times but on the occasions that we *do* drink we strongly reinvigorate the triggers relating to the circumstances. We strengthen triggers relating to the time, to the particular location and to certain people, but we also strengthen some universal triggers: the sight of alcohol and the smell of alcohol. We don't just strengthen the triggers associated with Friday after work we also strengthen them for any time we smell or see (or see in pictures, or imagine) alcohol. Each Friday we strengthen these triggers further and soon we find ourselves justifying drinking on "special occasions" outside the boundary we set. Once this happens then we strengthen more and more triggers and soon our reward system resumes its runaway state. We are no more able to keep our drinking to within certain bounds than we were before, and sooner or later the triggers once again overtake our ability to manage them.

If we try to return to moderate drinking *without* holding ourselves to strict boundaries then we bring all of our main drinking triggers back up to their former strength very quickly indeed and it takes only a few drinking sessions for our reward system to return to its runaway state.

But reinvigorating our drinking triggers is not the only consequence of relapse, something else happens that is even more serious. While we drank heavily then our brain adapted to offset alcohol impairment by accelerating processing speed and raising readiness to respond to an emergency. These changes kept us safer while we drank but they left us anxious and depressed when we were sober. Drinking to relieve the symptoms of alcohol-tolerance is what trapped us into the vicious cycle of addiction. All of the changes that come with alcohol-tolerance reverse back to normal levels once we are alcohol-free again for a period. But when our brain function is once again impaired by frequently high blood/alcohol levels then our brain recognises that it has met these conditions before and it reinstates all the remedial measures that were previously effective. All of the changes that our brain made when becoming alcohol-tolerant are put back in place. Our mood is lowered, our brain is speeded up, and anxiety and depression return. But this time the change doesn't happen over the months or years that it took the first time, this time it happens within days.

We can no more control our drinking after a period of abstinence than we could before and this is thoroughly proven to us if we try. Within only a few days of resuming drinking we are thrown right back to the same state of fear, anxiety, restlessness and hopelessness that had previously taken years to accumulate. When our brain reinstates the defensive measures of alcohol-tolerance then we once again drink to relieve the symptoms of drinking and this fixes our addiction back into place. Once we do this then our descent into hopelessness continues from where it left off. If however we have the strength of mind to stop after only having a couple of drinks then our brain *does not* re-implement the changes of alcohol-tolerance. Taking a few drinks and then returning to abstinence re-strengthens a few triggers and makes us feel jittery the next day but that is all. That is all except for the intense feeling of failure.

The consistent advice given to people that have relapsed is that we should get straight back up and give it another go but the emotional consequences of relapse are crushing. It feels like complete and total failure. We have failed in front of those close to us, we have failed in front of our peers, and we have failed ourselves. All I had to do was one simple thing, something that everyone else in the world seems able to do quite easily. But somehow I could not do it and the position seemed to be more hopeless than ever. Not only had I failed myself I had failed everyone else and it seemed that I really was the hopeless alcoholic that people thought I was. Relapse is a complete collapse of self-worth. Under these conditions it is extremely difficult to follow the advice given... to get back up and start again. The monstrous sense of failure makes me want to do one thing, and one thing only... to get drunk. But if I do this then I will quickly recommit myself onto a course into destruction. If I pursue this course then I will again have to sink to a terrible low before again reaching that point that point of desperation that powers my need to escape. This could take months and have untold consequences. What I need to do is stand myself up again quickly before I make things even worse.

I needed to radically change how I perceived relapse so that it did not itself become a barrier to recovery. The way to do this was to abandon the expectation that I should become alcohol-free at my first attempt, and I should do this because it is ridiculous. There is always a progression of steps we go through before we are able to achieve long-term sobriety, and we fail them, some of them many times, before we gain a long-lasting freedom. Before I even tried to stop I had already failed on many, many occasions to limit the amount I drank. I also drank on occasions I intended not to, I drank on days I said I wouldn't, and I failed to not drink for set periods of time. Each failure taught me that the challenge was sterner than I thought. I gradually improved my ability to remain alcohol-free, and I did this on the back of successive failures.

Nobody ever says "Day 1 again, and it was totally worth it!" Relapse feels dreadful, like complete failure, but it shouldn't because it isn't even unusual; it is the norm. Stopping drinking isn't like a test that we pass or fail; it is like a skill that we learn. When I was learning to ride a bike I often fell. It wasn't what I was trying to achieve, I didn't do it on purpose, and I didn't fall because I wasn't trying hard enough. I fell because I lacked the skill not to. But I wasn't thrown into despair when I fell off and I wasn't because there was no expectation that I would be successful at my first attempt. Sure, I got some scrapes, and my pride was a bit hurt, but I didn't give up and walk away, I got up and tried again. Stopping drinking is also a skill to be learned, but for some perverse reason the expectation is quite different. The expectation is that we should succeed at the first attempt, but this defies reason and it ignores reality. It is so unrealistic it is almost absurd. Very few people get sober at their first attempt and those that do suffer countless failures prior to their even trying. We don't just get one chance at learning to ride a bike and if we did then nobody would ever succeed. If we were expected to successfully ride a bike at our first attempt then almost everyone would fail and feel dejected. But that is not the assumption. We are told that we will learn to ride a bike if we practise and persist. So we keep trying until we succeed. We should apply that same expectation to stopping drinking. We learn to ride a bike by advancing through successive failures and this also how we learn to stop drinking. At first we are insecure and wobbly on a bike. We fall many times before we will even lift our feet fully to the pedals, and even when we do we may still fall at any moment. But with practice we become more secure, and more confident. Eventually we are able to go freely, in any direction we like, and we barely need to think about it at all. We learn to ride a bike through successive failures, but eventually we become able to do so with nearly no effort and this is also how we stop drinking. We improve our ability with application and practice. Relapse, if it happens, isn't some heinous failure. It isn't what we were trying to achieve but we had not yet gained sufficient skill to avoid it. It isn't failure, it is education, and if we drink again then it is a necessary learning step that will allow us to succeed later.

Even though it feels like it at the time we are not right back at the beginning and starting all over again. Nothing is lost and we are *not* back at the start of recovery. We still know everything that we have learned thus far and we just learned something new. A relapse does not put us back at the beginning of our recovery; it is a pause in the journey and no more. In fact, as long as we learn from the event, it advances us. If you have just relapsed then you should remember that the problem hasn't got worse because of it, the problem has not changed. You are still an alcoholic. You still can't limit or control your drinking, and continued drinking will drive you further along the downward spiral into despair. It had to stop, and it still has to stop. The problem is unchanged. What *is* changed though is your ability to succeed. Recovery is built on the experience of near-misses and relapse and it is these that allow us to advance into a life without alcohol.

I had to fall in order to learn to ride a bike, and stopping drinking sometimes requires similar learning. We often count days since we last drank as the measurement of success but it is important to recognise just what this is, or more significantly, what it is not.

The number of sober days we have accumulated only means the number of consecutive days of abstinence. But this is not a measure of recovery; it is a measure of sobriety. Recovery is not determined by the number of days since my last drink, it is measured by gains to my mental wellness, and the two can be quite independent of each other. If I drink again then my length of continuous sobriety is lost but my recovery isn't. I don't have to go right back to the beginning and start the process all over again. When I fell off the bicycle I wasn't put back at the start of learning how to ride, I was exactly as far advanced along that path as I was when I fell. Nothing was lost other that a bit of pride and skin. Everything that had been learned was still learned, and because of this fall I would do better at my next attempt. Relapse while trying to stop drinking is precisely like this; we are not put back at the start of recovery. We still know everything that we have learned thus far and we have just learned something new. If we have just confirmed that we can never regain control of our drinking then this is an invaluable lesson that is well worth the cost in hurt pride. A relapse does not put me back at the beginning of my recovery. In fact, as long as I learn from the experience, it advances me.

Stopping drinking is difficult and I didn't fully understand how difficult it was until I tried it in earnest. As I started out I was completely unaware of the full ferocity of cravings or all the ways that my mind would try to trick me into drinking again. I only discovered this as I went along and sometimes they caught me out and I drank. But relapse isn't failure, it is education. A relapse didn't make the problem worse, the problem remained unchanged. What *had* changed though was my ability to overcome it.

Nobody ever said we only get one chance at getting sober and we don't; we get as many as it takes, and it took many failures before I began to even try. All of these were building a better understanding of the problem, and relapse is learning too. Once I recognised that I couldn't control my drinking then I bit the bullet and tried to stop completely. But only a few succeed at their first attempt because most still have more learning to do and I was no different. While we can take some knowledge from books, or from other people in recovery, there are some things that I did not fully believe without first-hand experience, and the idea that I could never drink again was one of these. So I drank again to find out and when I did so I discovered that the books were right, and what people had said was right, and I had now confirmed it for myself, again! If relapse was the price I paid for fully learning this then it was worth it.

The experience of relapse was desperately uncomfortable, but like falling when trying to ride a bike this fall meant that I would do better at my next attempt, so I tried to find the lesson and move on again. We don't need to possess some rare talent to stop drinking, what we need is to keep learning so that we can continue to make progress. If we relapsed then we did so because on that occasion the urgency of a craving exceeded our resolve to resist it; so identify the issue. Was the problem failing at a big craving? Or was it a failure of resolve? Or did I start doing something I should not have, or wasn't ready for yet? I did not relapse without a cause, so I shouldn't simply dismiss it as not having tried hard enough; I have to identify what I could have done that would have prevented it, and then include that in my routine.

Regardless of how long I remain sober I am never completely free from the possibility of relapse and recovery from alcoholism should be regarded as bringing the condition into remission rather than achieving a cure. If I ever think that I have beaten addiction and can have "just one" then I will soon discover to my dismay that my drinking is again completely beyond my control. I can stop drinking and alter the condition so that it no longer interferes with my life but I can't remove my addiction completely; the drinking triggers are still there and they always will be. So too is the inability to form proper alcohol-avoiding triggers. In this respect I am never completely cured because the roots of alcoholism remain in my reward system forever. If I ever drink again then I will re-invigorate the triggers I acted on, and if I continue to drink then alcohol-tolerance will quickly re-establish itself. I will soon find myself exactly back in the desperate position that I was before. This is not something that sometimes happens; it is something that *always* happens.

Relapse is an awful experience, so learn its lesson and move on. Identify the gap in your armour, attend to it, and get back on your way again.

Do something!

This book has laid out the principal tools of recovery but it has done so in a quite specific way. It identified the core challenges of addiction; overcoming cravings, managing resolve, defeating self-sabotage, biased memory, and adverse emotions. It showed how each of these operates entirely automatically in the sense that we can't directly prevent their action. It shows what they are doing, how to recognise their operation, and what remedial actions we can take. Explaining this reveals what we need to actively push back against and how. It described the tools we can use to counter these challenges, but it also showed why each is effective and this is important, because if I know that some remedial action will be effective then I will work harder at applying it. Every action suggested in this book has a clear therapeutic purpose and this takes the guesswork out of recovery and eliminates wasted effort. It also provides a pathway to succeed. At each step it shows what will help and why that action will work, and the key word here is action. Recovery is not a passive process and throughout this book there is one phrase that occurs more than any other and that is "*do something*".

I can't sit around and wait for someone else to fix this problem because nobody is going to, nor are they able to. I am the only person that will lift a drink to my mouth, and if that is what I want to do then nobody is able stop me. But equally I am the only person that can prevent this from happening. The actions required are not for others to take; they are mine and mine alone. I can use other people for inspiration, guidance, experience, and expertise, and I can use them to lift my resolve when it is flagging, but only I can do what is needed to recover. But not only am I the only one that can bring about my recovery, I am also the only barrier to it. Nothing and nobody else makes me want to pick up drink, I manufacture that between my own ears, and nothing and nobody else has the means to prevent me from drinking. I am responsible for my own recovery. I am the only one that can do this, and I am the only one preventing me from succeeding.

This book is not the most exciting piece of quit-lit you could read, and it does not attempt to be that. This book is a manual, not a novel. It has laid out a pathway to recovery and described the tools that will be effective, but all this is worthless while it remains on these pages. Do something. Start where you are with what you have and take it from there. Keep trying the things that should work. Keep doing the things that help, drop the ones that don't, and then move onto the next one that might. But at all times keep going, because progress is made in small increments. It may not be obvious that it is happening, but it is.

The effort involved in becoming well reduces as we become more accomplished at using the tools that help us, but the challenge is a stern one. I am driven into addiction by two key characteristics: I want more of the good stuff, and I want it now. This is what tipped my reward system into a runaway state and this is what set me on a course into disaster. But these two characteristics are precisely the opposite of what is required in recovery. The properties of my mind that conspire to make me drink are the same ones that diminish my ability to stop, indeed, addiction and lacking the means to stop are probably the same thing. I have to work actively to do what I lack naturally. If I am to stop drinking and to stay stopped then I have to deny myself something *now* because it will help me *later*. But this is a ridiculously difficult thing to achieve because it requires me to act against my very nature, and this is my Achilles heel. In order to become well I have to do something now, that I'm not motivated to do, in order to gain some benefit later, which I don't much care about. What causes my addiction also impedes my recovery and I need to learn this well. In order to recover I have to overcome me.

My mind lies to me about alcohol and I have no direct way of preventing that from happening. My task is to recognise the lies as they come and then counteract them by wit or force of will. We never get ahead of the curve on this, it is always reactive. I have to recognise each lie as it comes; be it a craving, a self-sabotaging idea, or a memory, and I have to recognise it as incorrect and reject it. I have to notice when my mind is doing something unwanted and then take some specific and deliberate action to counter it. It is a ridiculously difficult thing to do and it is even more difficult because there are so many individual deceptions to confront, tools to apply, and disciplines to master. But difficult is not impossible.

At first my recovery was chaotic and brittle. There were so many different things happening all at the same time and all needed some action on my part. I missed a lot of them. While I was working on one issue then I would miss another until its effect became so big that I suddenly needed to switch focus to deal with it. But improvement was steady. Once through withdrawal then the cravings slowly dropped in intensity and managing resolve and self-sabotage became the next skills I needed to concentrate on. When I mastered these then managing my emotional state became the main challenge. Every day was progress. Every day the impact of alcoholism on my daily life grew less intrusive as my means to promptly deal with its issues improved. The problem kept changing and I kept expanding my skill-set to match that change. I didn't immediately do everything right, I couldn't, I needed to learn and to practice, and often that meant being unsuccessful. I had to check what I was doing, adjust it and try again. In time I mastered more and more of the disciplines required and my recovery became more robust. But this took time and time is the very thing I am ill-equipped to tolerate. It was hard to maintain focus over a long time-scale and that is why staying engaged with a recovery community was absolutely essential to me. I needed connection to people that would reaffirm that my course was correct, remind me I have to do things to stay well, top-up my resolve, and to encourage me to keep going.

I didn't get it right first time, every time, but I slowly got better at managing my recovery. As my self-awareness grew, and I repeatedly acted to counteract a specific challenge, then these actions themselves began to become automatic. The aim is not immediate perfection; that is never going to happen, the aim is incremental improvement. This isn't what I want to hear because I am inherently impatient for results, but I had to train myself to accept it because this challenge takes time to overcome and there is no other way. If I want the result then this is the path.

Recovery isn't passive; it requires me to do things at every turn. At each problem I have to do something. I have to recognise the issue, know what will correct it, and then do it. There is some advice often given in recovery: "this too shall pass" but this is sometimes the worst advice for an alcoholic. This tells me to sit and endure some discomfort because it will be better later, but I don't care about later! If I am sitting with a problem then sitting with it will make it persist, but if I *do something* then I can *make* it go away. The path forward is never doing nothing, because doing nothing changes nothing. I do not change the way my mind works by letting unwanted mental processes go unchallenged. I change the way my mind works by repeatedly correcting the unwanted thinking. My brain does not learn new ways without new actions, so sitting and waiting achieves nothing; I need to act to change it. This is how I progress.

The traditional wisdom is that "A leopard can't change its spots" and while this inflexibility may be a true of leopards it is not true of us. We *can* change, but we do not change by being passive. We cannot wait for recovery to come to us. We have to do the things that will make those changes and we have to make those changes because untreated alcoholism is unsurvivable. No matter how bad it is now it will only get worse if we don't confront it. Do something. Do something now. Make it stop.

Also by David Horry

Lying Minds: An Insider's Guide to Alcoholism

Alcoholics are not damaged, faulty, or broken, and we aren't bad or weak people, we are deceived: deceived by our own minds. This book explains how our mind becomes deceived by alcohol 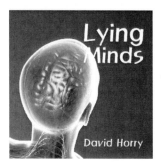 and how it changes our motivation, emotions, memory and thinking. It explains why we can never safely drink again, and the deeper truth... that we never could in the first place, we just didn't know it.

"Lying Minds" shows you what the problem is, and "Make it Stop" shows you what to do about it.

Made in United States
North Haven, CT
06 July 2022

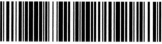

20997739R00126